T0294609

PAIN MEDICINE
A CASE-BASED LEARNING SERIES

The Ankle and Foot

Other books in this series:

The Spine
9780323756365

The Shoulder and Elbow
9780323758772

The Hip and Pelvis
9780323762977

The Knee
9780323762588

Headache and Facial Pain
9780323834568

The Wrist and Hand
9780323834537

The Chest Wall and Abdomen
9780323846882

PAIN MEDICINE
A CASE-BASED LEARNING SERIES

The Ankle and Foot

STEVEN D. WALDMAN, MD, JD

ELSEVIER

Elsevier
1600 John F. Kennedy Blvd.
Ste 1800
Philadelphia, PA 19103-2899

PAIN MEDICINE: A CASE-BASED LEARNING SERIES   ISBN: 978-0-323-87038-2
THE ANKLE AND FOOT

Copyright © 2023 by Elsevier, Inc. All rights reserved.

Executive Content Strategist: Michael Houston
Content Development Specialist: Jeannine Carrado/Laura Klein
Director, Content Development: Ellen Wurm-Cutter
Publishing Services Manager: Shereen Jameel
Senior Project Manager: Karthikeyan Murthy
Design Direction: Amy Buxton

Printed in India.

Last digit is the print number: 9 8 7 6 5 4 3 2 1

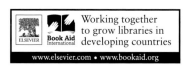

Working together to grow libraries in developing countries

www.elsevier.com • www.bookaid.org

It's Harder Than It Looks
MAKING THE CASE FOR CASE-BASED LEARNING

For the sake of full disclosure, I was one of those guys. You know, the ones who wax poetic about how hard it is to teach our students how to do procedures. Let me tell you, teaching folks how to do epidurals on women in labor certainly takes its toll on the coronary arteries. It's true, I am amazing ... I am great ... I have nerves of steel. Yes, I could go on like this for hours ... but you have heard it all before. But, it's again that time of year when our new students sit eagerly before us, full of hope and dreams ... and that harsh reality comes slamming home ... it is a lot harder to teach beginning medical students "doctoring" than it looks.

A few years ago, I was asked to teach first-year medical and physician assistant students how to take a history and perform a basic physical exam. In my mind this should be easy, no big deal, I won't have to do much more than show up. After all, I was the guy who wrote that amazing book on physical diagnosis. After all, I had been teaching medical students, residents, and fellows how to do highly technical (and dangerous, I might add) interventional pain management procedures since seemingly right after the Civil War. Seriously, it was no big deal ... I could do it in my sleep ... with one arm tied behind my back ... blah ... blah ... blah.

For those of you who have had the privilege of teaching "doctoring," you already know what I am going to say next. *It's harder than it looks!* Let me repeat this to disabuse any of you who, like me, didn't get it the first time. *It is harder than it looks!* I only had to meet with my first-year medical and physician assistant students a couple of times to get it through my thick skull: **It really is harder than it looks**. In case you are wondering, the reason that our students look back at us with those blank, confused, bored, and ultimately dismissive looks is simple: They lack context. That's right, they lack the context to understand what we are talking about.

It's really that simple ... or hard ... depending on your point of view or stubbornness, as the case may be. To understand why context is king, you have to look only as far as something as basic as the Review of Systems. The Review of Systems is about as basic as it gets, yet why is it so perplexing to our students? Context. I guess it should come as no surprise to anyone that the student is completely lost when you talk about ... let's say ... the "constitutional" portion of the Review of Systems, without the context of what a specific constitutional finding, say a fever or chills, might mean to a patient. If you tell the student that you need to ask about fever, chills, and the other "constitutional" stuff and you take it no further, you might as well be talking about the International Space

Station. Just save your breath; it makes absolutely no sense to your students. Yes, they want to please, so they will memorize the elements of the Review of Systems, but that is about as far as it goes. On the other hand, if you present the case of Jannette Patton, a 28-year-old first-year medical resident with a fever and headache, you can see the lights start to come on. By the way, this is what Jannette looks like, and as you can see, Jannette is sicker than a dog. This, at its most basic level, is what *Case-Based Learning* is all about.

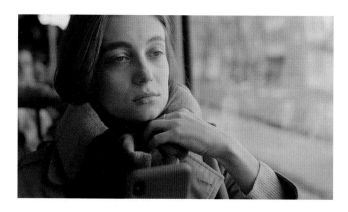

I would like to tell you that, smart guy that I am, I immediately saw the light and became a convert to *Case-Based Learning*. But truth be told, it was COVID-19 that really got me thinking about *Case-Based Learning*. Before the COVID-19 pandemic, I could just drag the students down to the med/surg wards and walk into a patient room and riff. Everyone was a winner. For the most part, the patients loved to play along and thought it was cool. The patient and the bedside was all I needed to provide the context that was necessary to illustrate what I was trying to teach—the "why headache and fever don't mix" kind of stuff. Had COVID-19 not rudely disrupted my ability to teach at the bedside, I suspect that you would not be reading this *Preface*, as I would not have had to write it. Within a very few days after the COVID-19 pandemic hit, my days of bedside teaching disappeared, but my students still needed context. This got me focused on how to provide the context they needed. The answer was, of course, *Case-Based Learning*. What started as a desire to provide context . . . because it really was **harder than it looked** . . . led me to begin work on this eight-volume *Case-Based Learning* textbook series. What you will find within these volumes are a bunch of fun, real-life cases that help make each patient come alive for the student. These cases provide the contextual teaching points that make it easy for the teacher to explain why, when Jannette's chief complaint is, *"My head is killing me and I've got a fever,"* it is a big deal.

Have fun!

Steven D. Waldman, MD, JD
Spring 2021

ACKNOWLEDGMENTS

A very special thanks to my editors, Michael Houston, PhD, Jeannine Carrado, and Karthikeyan Murthy, for all their hard work and perseverance in the face of disaster. Great editors such as Michael, Jeannine, and Karthikeyan make their authors look great, for they not only understand how to bring the Three Cs of great writing...Clarity + Consistency + Conciseness...to the author's work, but unlike me, they can actually punctuate and spell!

Steven D. Waldman, MD, JD

P.S. ...Sorry for all the ellipses, guys!

CONTENTS

Ryan Rostov

A 52-Year-Old Male With Right Ankle Pain

- Learn the common causes of ankle pain.
- Develop an understanding of the unique anatomy of the ankle joint.
- Develop an understanding of the causes of ankle joint arthritis.
- Learn the clinical presentation of osteoarthritis of the ankle joint.
- Learn how to use physical examination to identify pathology of the ankle joint.
- Develop an understanding of the treatment options for osteoarthritis of the ankle joint.
- Learn the appropriate testing options to help diagnose osteoarthritis of the ankle joint.
- Learn to identify red flags in patients who present with ankle pain.
- Develop an understanding of the role in interventional pain management in the treatment of ankle pain.

Ryan Rostov

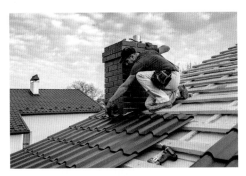

Ryan Rostov is a 52-year-old roofer with the chief complaint of, "My right ankle is killing me." Ryan went on to say that he wouldn't have bothered coming in, but he was getting to where he was having a harder and harder time walking on roofs with a steep pitch. "Doctor, it's getting to where I am afraid to work on some of these steep roofs. It's not a height sort of thing, nothing like that. It's just when I flex my right ankle to walk down the roof, I get a sharp pain. I am afraid it will hit when I am not expecting it, and I will lose my footing. I am not interested in falling off the roofs of some of the McMansions, if you know what I mean." I asked Ryan if he had anything like this happen before. He shook his head and responded, "Just the usual aches that a guy my age comes to expect. You can't work all day as a roofer and not have some pain. On some days I go up and down a ladder 100 times. Usually, I just take a couple of Motrin and use a heating pad. That will usually set me right after a day or so. What worries me this time is that this damn right ankle is hurting all the time. Especially, like I said, when I'm coming down a roof. I can live with the aching, but it's that sharp pain that scares me. I'm pretty tough and I really like what I do. There's a start and a finish to it. The roof leaks, I put on a roof, no more leaks. Kind of like being a doctor! But this ankle pain has me worried because if I don't work, I don't eat. In my younger days, when I should have been saving, I was playing. I really need to work if I ever want to retire, which I don't yet! So help me get this ankle tuned up."

I asked Ryan about any antecedent trauma, and he shook his head no. "Doc, this kind of snuck up on me. At first, my ankle had this deep ache that would get better with some Motrin and rest. Over time, the Motrin has just about quit working. But, like I said, I gotta work." I asked Ryan what made his pain worse, and he replied, "The steeper the pitch, the worse the ankle."

I asked Ryan to point with one finger to show me where it hurt the most. He grabbed his right ankle and said, "Doc, I can't really point to one place because it kind of hurts all over. Although, by the end of the day, the front of the ankle is the worst. And you know, Doc, the crazy thing is, sometimes I feel like the ankle is popping." I asked if he had any fever or chills, and he shook his head no. I continued, "What about steroids? Did you ever take any cortisone or drugs like that?" Ryan again shook his head no, then said, "You know me, I'm not one for taking pills. Pills and roofing really don't mix."

On physical examination, Ryan was afebrile. His respirations were 16, and his pulse was 74 and regular. His blood pressure was slightly elevated at 122/74. His head, eyes, ears, nose, throat (HEENT) exam was normal, as was his cardio-pulmonary examination. His thyroid was normal. His abdominal examination revealed no abnormal mass or organomegaly. There was no costovertebral angle (CVA) tenderness. There was no peripheral edema. His low back examination was unremarkable. I did a rectal exam, which revealed no mass and a normal prostate. Visual inspection of the right ankle revealed no cutaneous lesions or obvious tumor. The ankle was cool to touch. Palpation of the right ankle revealed mild diffuse tenderness, with a mild effusion (Fig. 1.1). There was tenderness at the anterior aspect of the ankle joint. There was mild crepitus, but I did not appreciate any popping or joint instability. Range of motion of the ankle joint was decreased, with pain exacerbated with flexion, extension, eversion, and inversion of the ankle. The anterior drawer test for anterior talofibular ligament instability was negative (Fig. 1.2). The left ankle examination was normal, as was examination of his other major joints, other than some mild osteoarthritis in the

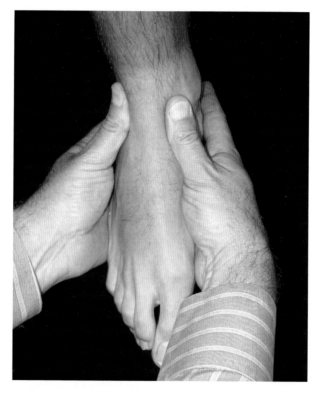

Fig. 1.1   Palpation of the ankle joint. (From Waldman S. *Physical Diagnosis of Pain: An Atlas of Signs and Symptoms*. ed. 4. Philadelphia: Elsevier; 2021 [Fig. 262-1].)

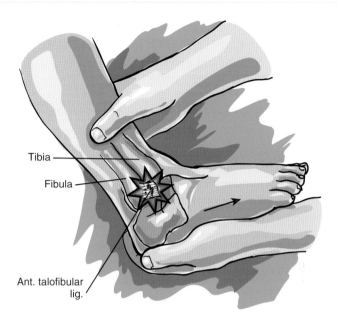

Fig. 1.2 The anterior drawer test for anterior talofibular ligament insufficiency. (From Waldman S. *Physical Diagnosis of Pain: An Atlas of Signs and Symptoms*. ed. 4. Philadelphia: Elsevier; 2021 [Fig. 264-1].)

right hand. A careful neurologic examination of the upper and lower extremities revealed no evidence of peripheral or entrapment neuropathy, and the deep tendon reflexes were normal.

Key Clinical Points—What's Important and What's Not

THE HISTORY

- No history of acute trauma
- No history of previous significant ankle pain
- No fever or chills
- Gradual onset of ankle pain with exacerbation of pain with ankle use
- Popping sensation in the right ankle
- Sleep disturbance
- Intermittent sharp pain in the anterior ankle with flexion of the joint

THE PHYSICAL EXAMINATION

- Patient is afebrile
- Normal visual inspection of ankle other than mild effusion

- Palpation of right ankle reveals diffuse tenderness
- Decreased range of motion of the ankle joint; pain exacerbated with ankle flexion, extension, eversion, and inversion
- No increased temperature of right ankle
- Crepitus to palpation (see Fig. 1.1)
- Negative anterior drawer test (see Fig. 1.2)

OTHER FINDINGS OF NOTE

- Normal HEENT examination
- Normal cardiovascular examination
- Normal pulmonary examination
- Normal abdominal examination
- No peripheral edema
- Normal upper and lower extremity neurologic examination, motor and sensory examination
- Examination of other joints was normal

 ## What Tests Would You Like to Order?

The following tests were ordered:
- Plain radiographs of the right ankle

TEST RESULTS

The anterior to posterior (AP) and lateral radiographs of the ankle joint indicate severe ankle arthritis with reduced joint space, anterior osteophytes, and sclerosis of the articular surfaces consistent with osteoarthritis (Fig. 1.3).

 ## Clinical Correlation—Putting It All Together

What is the diagnosis?
- Osteoarthritis of the right ankle joint

The Science Behind the Diagnosis
ANATOMY OF THE JOINTS OF THE ANKLE

The ankle is a hinge-type articulation among the distal tibia, the two malleoli, and the talus (Fig. 1.4). The articular surface is covered with hyaline cartilage, which is susceptible to arthritis. The joint is surrounded by a dense capsule, which helps strengthen the ankle. The joint capsule is lined with a synovial

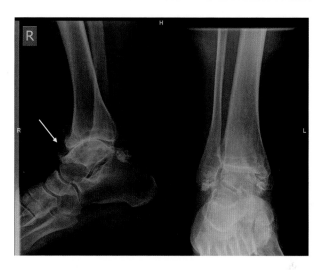

Fig. 1.3 Anteroposterior and lateral radiographs of an ankle joint indicating severe ankle arthritis with a large anterior osteophyte *(white arrow)*. (From Adukia V, Mangwani J, Issac R, et al. Current concepts in the management of ankle arthritis. *J Clin Orthop Trauma*. 2020;11(3):388–398 [Fig. 1].)

membrane that attaches to the articular cartilage. The ankle joint is innervated by the deep peroneal and tibial nerves. The major ligaments of the ankle joint include the deltoid, anterior talofibular, calcaneofibular, and posterior talofibular ligaments, which provide the majority of strength to the ankle joint. The muscles of the ankle and their attaching tendons are susceptible to trauma and to wear and tear from overuse and misuse. There are a number of arteries that traverse the joint that can provide sources of bleeding when performing intraarticular injection of the ankle (Fig. 1.5).

THE CLINICAL SYNDROME

Arthritis of the ankle is a common condition. The ankle joint is susceptible to the development of arthritis from various conditions that can damage the joint cartilage (Fig. 1.6). Osteoarthritis is the most common form of arthritis that results in ankle pain; rheumatoid arthritis and posttraumatic arthritis are also frequent causes of ankle pain. Less common causes include collagen vascular diseases, infection, villonodular synovitis, and Lyme disease (Fig. 1.7). Acute infectious arthritis is usually accompanied by significant systemic symptoms, including fever and malaise, and should be easily recognized; it is treated with culture and antibiotics rather than injection therapy. Collagen vascular disease generally manifests as polyarthropathy rather than monoarthropathy limited to the ankle joint, although ankle pain secondary to collagen vascular disease responds exceedingly well to the treatment modalities described here.

A

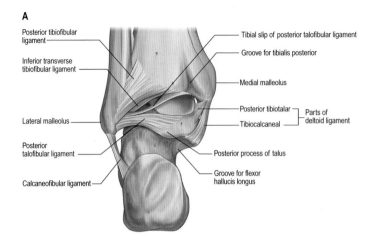

B

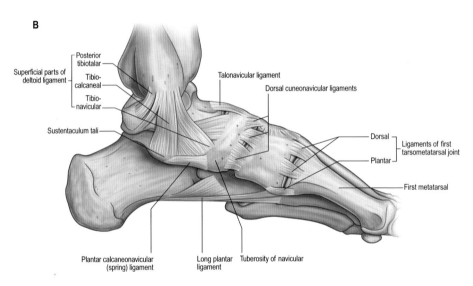

Fig. 1.4   The ankle is a hinge-type articulation among the distal tibia, the two malleoli, and the talus. (A) Posterior view. (B) Medial aspect. (From Standring S. *Grays Anatomy: The Anatomic Basis of Clinical Practice*. ed. 42. Philadelphia: Elsevier; 2021 [Fig. 79-14].)

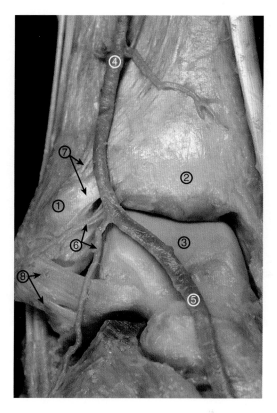

Fig. 1.5 Anatomic dissection showing the varying course of the anterior tibial artery (lateral deviation). *1*, Lateral malleolus; *2*, tibia; *3*, talus; *4*, anterior tibial artery; *5*, dorsalis pedis artery; *6*, anterior malleolar artery; *7*, anterior tibiofibular ligament; *8*, anterior talofibular ligament. (From Golanó P, Vega J, Pérez-Carro L, Götzens V. Ankle anatomy for the arthroscopist. Part I: the portals. *Foot Ankle Clin.* 2006;11:253–273.)

SIGNS AND SYMPTOMS

Most patients complain of pain localized around the ankle and distal lower extremity. Activity makes the pain worse, whereas rest and heat provide some relief. The pain is constant and is characterized as aching; it may interfere with sleep. Some patients complain of a grating or popping sensation with use of the joint, and crepitus may be present on physical examination.

In addition to pain, patients with arthritis of the ankle often experience a gradual decrease in functional ability because of reduced ankle range of motion that makes simple everyday tasks, such as walking and climbing stairs and ladders, quite difficult (Fig. 1.8). With continued disuse, muscle wasting may occur, and a frozen ankle secondary to adhesive capsulitis may develop.

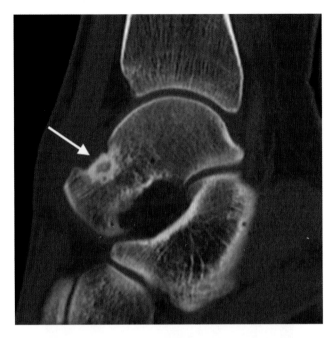

Fig. 1.6 Computed tomography of an osteoid osteoma of the talar neck with typical perifocal sclerosis and a central nidus. (From Toepfer A. Tumors of the foot and ankle—a review of the principles of diagnostics and treatment. *Fuß & Sprunggelenk*. 2017;15(2):82—96 [Fig. 7].)

TESTING

Plain radiographs are indicated in all patients who present with ankle pain (Fig. 1.9). Computed tomography scanning may help further clarify the diagnosis and identify other occult bony pathology (see Fig. 1.6). Magnetic resonance imaging (MRI) and ultrasound imaging of the ankle are indicated in the case of trauma, if the diagnosis is in question, or if an occult mass or tumor is suspected (Figs. 1.10 and 1.11). Radionuclide imaging may further clarify the source of the patient's pain (Fig. 1.12). Based on the patient's clinical presentation, additional testing may be warranted, including a complete blood count, comprehensive metabolic profile, erythrocyte sedimentation rate, and antinuclear antibody testing.

DIFFERENTIAL DIAGNOSIS

Lumbar radiculopathy may mimic the pain and disability of arthritis of the ankle; however, results of the ankle examination are negative (Box 1.1). Bursitis and tendinitis of the ankle and entrapment neuropathies, such as tarsal tunnel syndrome, may also confuse the diagnosis; both of these conditions may coexist

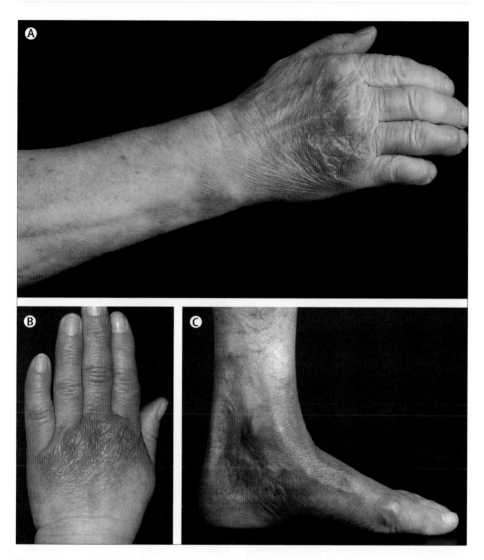

Fig. 1.7 Lyme disease is an uncommon cause of ankle pain that must be included in the differential diagnosis. Acrodermatitis chronic atrophicans is an uncommon cutaneous manifestation of European Lyme disease and is typically located on the extensor sites of extremities: (A) ulnar and hand lesions, (B) bluish-red lesion on the back of a patient's hand and waxy appearance of the skin of fingers, and (C) lesions on a patient's left foot and lower leg. Reprinted with permission from Elsevier (from Gerold Stanek, Gary P Wormser, Jeremy Gray, Franc Strle, Lyme borreliosis. *The Lancet.* 2012;379(9814): 461–473 [Fig. 5].)

with arthritis of the ankle (Fig. 1.13 and Box 1.2). Primary and metastatic tumors of the distal tibia and fibula and spine, as well as occult fractures, may also manifest in a manner similar to arthritis of the ankle.

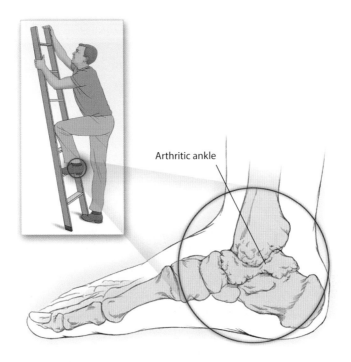

Arthritic ankle

Fig. 1.8 Arthritis of the ankle is often made worse with activity. (From Waldman S. *Atlas of Common Pain Syndromes*. ed. 4. Philadelphia: Elsevier; 2019 [Fig. 121-1].)

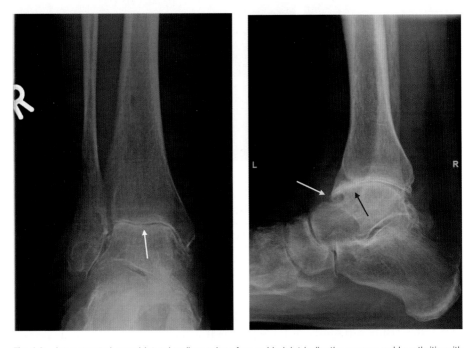

Fig. 1.9 Anteroposterior and lateral radiographs of an ankle joint indicating severe ankle arthritis with reduced joint space *(white arrow)*, anterior osteophytes *(yellow arrow)*, and sclerosis *(red arrow)*. (From Adukia V, Mangwani J, Issac R, et al. Current concepts in the management of ankle arthritis. *J Clin Orthop Trauma*. 2020;11(3):388–398 [Fig. 2].)

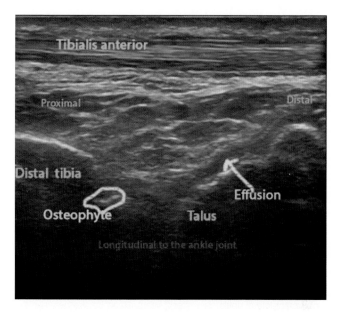

Fig. 1.10 Longitudinal ultrasound image of the ankle demonstrating findings consistent with osteo-arthritis. Note the osteophyte formation and effusion.

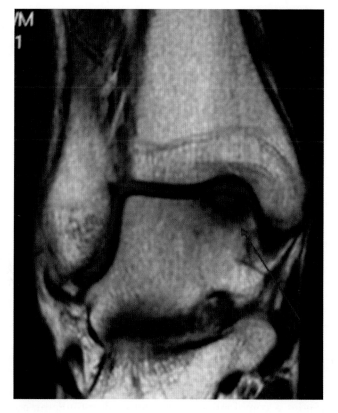

Fig. 1.11 Magnetic resonance imaging coronal view of an ankle showing an osteochondral defect *(red arrow)*. (From Adukia V, Mangwani J, Issac R, et al. Current concepts in the management of ankle arthritis. *J Clin Orthop Trauma.* 2020;11(3):388–398 [Fig. 3].)

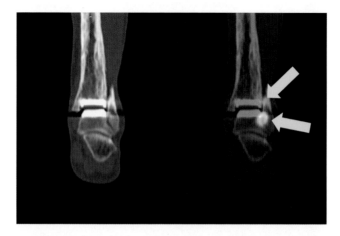

Fig. 1.12 This 59-year-old man had a surgical repair of a left ankle fracture 5 years ago. Hardware was removed from the joint and long bones 3 years later, and a total ankle replacement (TAR) was inserted. He has persistent lateral ankle pain after 2 years. Bone uptake between the prosthesis and the fibula appears to implicate impingement of the metal on the fibular cortex as the cause of his pain. (From Waldman LE, Scharf SC. Bone SPECT/CT of the spine, foot, and ankle: evaluation of surgical patients. *Semin Nucl Med*. 2017;47(6):639–646 [Fig. 6].)

BOX 1.1 ■ Differential Diagnosis of Ankle Pain

1. Osteoarthritis
2. Avulsion fracture
3. Intraarticular fracture
4. Stress fractures
5. Achilles tendinitis
6. Achilles bursitis
7. Bursitis
8. Ligamentous sprains
9. Ligamentous strains
10. Gout
11. Other crystal arthropathies
12. Psoriatic arthritis
13. Reactive arthritis
14. Rheumatoid arthritis
15. Septic arthritis
16. Osteochondritis dissecans
17. Anterior tarsal tunnel syndrome
18. Posterior tarsal tunnel syndrome
19. Lyme disease

TREATMENT

Initial treatment of the pain and functional disability associated with arthritis of the ankle includes a combination of nonsteroidal antiinflammatory drugs or

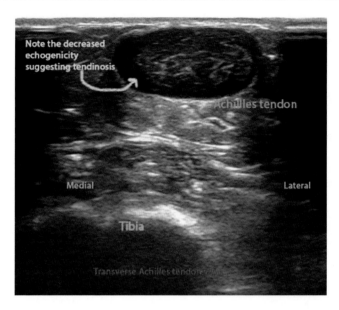

Fig. 1.13   Tendinopathy of the Achilles tendon is a common cause of ankle pain and may coexist with osteoarthritis of the ankle. Transverse ultrasound image of the Achilles tendon demonstrating tendinopathy.

BOX 1.2 ■ Painful Disorders of the Ankle and the Foot

Articular

Arthritis	RA, OA, PsA, gout
Toe disorders	Hallux valgus, hallux rigidus, hammer toe
Arch disorders	Pes planus, pes cavus

Periarticular

Cutaneous	Corn, callosity
Subcutaneous	RA nodules, tophi
	Ingrown toenail
Plantar fascia	Plantar fasciitis
	Plantar nodular fibromatosis
Tendons	Achilles tendinitis
	Achilles tendon rupture
	Tibialis posterior tenosynovitis
	Peroneal tenosynovitis
Bursae	Bunion, bunionette
	Retrocalcaneal, retroachilleal, and subcalcaneal bursitis
	Medial and lateral malleolar bursitis
Acute calcific periarthritis	Hydroxyapatite pseudopodagra (first MTP)

(Continued)

Osseous

Fracture (traumatic, stress)
Sesamoiditis
Neoplasm
Infection
Epiphysitis (osteochondritis)

Painful accessory ossicles

Second metatarsal head (Freiberg disease)
Navicular (Köhler disease)
Calcaneus (Sever disease)
Accessory navicular
Os trigonum (near talus)
Os intermetatarseum (first and second)

Neurologic

Tarsal tunnel syndrome
Interdigital (Morton) neuroma
Peripheral neuropathy
Radiculopathy (lumbar disk)

Vascular

Ischemic
Vasospastic disorder (Raynaud disease)
Cholesterol emboli with "purple toes"

Atherosclerosis, Buerger disease

Referred

Lumbosacral spine
Knee
Chronic regional pain syndrome I
Chronic regional pain syndrome II

Modified from Lawry G, Kreder H, Hawker G, et al. *Fam's Musculoskeletal Examination and Joint Injection Techniques*. ed. 2. Philadelphia: Mosby; 2010:89–101.

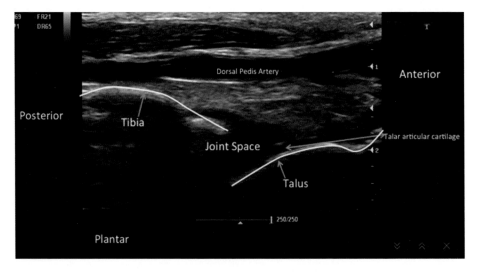

Fig. 1.14 Ultrasound-guided injection of the ankle joint.

cyclooxygenase-2 inhibitors and physical therapy. The local application of heat and cold may also be beneficial. Avoidance of repetitive activities that aggravate the patient's symptoms, as well as short-term immobilization of the ankle joint, may provide relief. For patients who do not respond to these treatment modalities, intraarticular injection of local anesthetic and steroid is a reasonable next step. Ultrasound needle guidance will improve the accuracy of needle placement and decrease the incidence of needle-related complications (Fig. 1.14). The injection of platelet-rich plasma and/or stem cells may reduce the pain and functional disability of ankle arthritis.

Physical modalities, including local heat and gentle range-of-motion exercises, should be introduced several days after the patient undergoes injection. Vigorous exercises should be avoided because they will exacerbate the patient's symptoms.

HIGH-YIELD TAKEAWAYS

- The patient is afebrile, making an acute infectious etiology (e.g., septic arthritis) unlikely.
- The patient's symptomatology is not the result of acute trauma but more likely the result of repetitive microtrauma that has damaged the joint over time.
- The patient's pain is diffuse rather than highly localized, as would be the case with a pathologic process such as Achilles tendinitis.
- The patient's symptoms are unilateral and only involve one joint, which is more suggestive of a local process rather than a systemic polyarthropathy.
- Plain radiographs will provide high-yield information regarding the bony contents of the joint, but ultrasound imaging and MRI will be more useful in identifying soft tissue pathology.

Suggested Readings

Repetto I, Biti B, Cerruti P, et al. Conservative treatment of ankle osteoarthritis: can platelet-rich plasma effectively postpone surgery? *J Foot Ankle Surg.* 2017;56(2): 362−365.

Robinson AHN, Keith T. Osteoarthritis of the ankle. *Orthop Trauma.* 2016;30(1):59−67.

Waldman SD. Arthritis and other abnormalities of the ankle joint. In: *Waldman's Comprehensive Atlas of Diagnostic Ultrasound of Painful Conditions.* Philadelphia: Wolters Kluwer; 2016:875−882.

Waldman SD. Arthritis pain of the ankle. In: *Atlas of Common Pain Syndromes.* ed. 4. Philadelphia: Elsevier; 2019:480−483.

Waldman SD. Functional anatomy of the ankle and foot. In: *Pain Review.* ed. 2. Philadelphia: Elsevier; 2017:149−150.

Waldman SD. Functional anatomy of the ankle and foot. In: *Physical Diagnosis of Pain: An Atlas of Signs and Symptoms.* ed. 4. Philadelphia: Elsevier; 2021:390−393.

Waldman SD. Intra-articular injection of the ankle joint. In: *Atlas of Pain Management Injection Techniques*. ed. 4. Philadelphia: Elsevier; 2017:587–589.

Waldman SD. Ultrasound-guided injection technique for intra-articular injection of the ankle joint. In: *Comprehensive Atlas of Ultrasound-Guided Pain Management Injection Techniques*. Philadelphia: Wolters Kluwer; 2020:1141–1146.

Waldman SD, Campbell RSD. Anatomy: special imaging considerations of the ankle and foot. In: *Imaging of Pain*. Philadelphia: Saunders; 2011:417–420.

Shirley McCain

A 62-Year-Old Dance Instructor With Right Foot Pain

LEARNING OBJECTIVES

- Learn the common causes of foot pain.
- Develop an understanding of the unique anatomy of the midtarsal joint.
- Develop an understanding of the causes of midtarsal joint arthritis.
- Learn the clinical presentation of osteoarthritis of the midtarsal joint.
- Learn how to use physical examination to identify pathology of the midtarsal joint.
- Develop an understanding of the treatment options for osteoarthritis of the midtarsal joint.
- Learn the appropriate testing options to help diagnose osteoarthritis of the midtarsal joint.
- Learn to identify red flags in patients who present with foot pain.
- Develop an understanding of the role in interventional pain management in the treatment of foot pain.

Shirley McCain

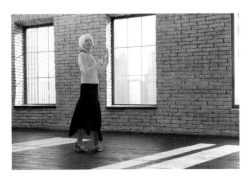

Shirley McCain is a 62-year-old dance instructor with the chief complaint of, "My right foot is killing me." Shirley went on to say that she wouldn't have bothered coming in, but, "It's getting harder and harder for me to teach my students. By the end of a class, I can barely stand up, let alone demon-strate a dance step." I asked Shirley if anything like this has happened before. She shook her head no, and said that she had been a dancer all her life and that she had always taken great care of her feet. "Doctor, I started out as a ballet dancer, which is really hard on the feet. I was a good dancer—but not good enough. Fortunately, very early on, I learned that I really enjoyed teaching. Unlike professional dance, your suc-cesses as a dance instructor are up close and personal. But I apologize, Doctor, I am rambling. What do you want to know? Oh, and one of my students said you could give me a cortisone shot to get my foot better. I really hope you can. I'm sorry, I guess coming to the doctor makes me nervous, and when I'm nervous I tend to chatter."

I asked Shirley about any antecedent trauma to the right foot. She thought about it for a minute, then said that she did sprain her foot many years ago when she was still an understudy with the ballet company. She went on to say that it was, in fact, that sprain that got her thinking about what she could do if she couldn't continue with ballet. "Doctor, I was young and thought it would last forever. It never entered my mind I would do anything other than be in the ballet. It took longer for my ankle to heal than I thought it would, so I picked up some part-time work teaching ballet to grade-school children. Who would have thought? I loved it, and I guess the rest is history. But there I go again. I'm so sorry, Doctor." I smiled and told Shirley that I was enjoying her story.

I then asked Shirley to point with one finger to show me where it hurt the most. She pointed to the top of her right foot and said, "Doc, it hurts right here, especially when I push off. Like when I do the cha-cha. You know, right, left, cha-cha-cha? When that right foot goes back, it really hurts." I asked if she had any fever or chills, and she shook her head no. I continued, "What about ste-roids? Did you ever take any cortisone or drugs like that?" Shirley again shook her head no. "Doctor, I am not one to take pills, but I need to do something because my foot soaks are not doing the trick."

On physical examination, Shirley was afebrile. Her respirations were 18, and her pulse was 74 and regular. Her blood pressure was normal at 122/74. Her head, eyes, ears, nose, throat (HEENT) exam was normal, as was her cardiopulmonary examination. Her thyroid was normal. Her abdominal examination revealed no abnormal mass or organomegaly. There was no costovertebral angle (CVA) tenderness. There was no peripheral edema. Her low back examination was unremarkable. Visual inspection of the right ankle and foot revealed no cutaneous lesions or abnormal mass. The area overlying the dorsum of the right ankle and foot was cool to touch, with no evidence of infection. Her dorsalis pedis pulse was 1+. Palpation of the right foot revealed mild diffuse tenderness, with no obvious effusion or point tenderness. I did not appreciate any popping or crepitus with movement of the foot and ankle. Dorsiflexion and plantar flexion of the right foot and ankle reproduced Shirley's pain. The left foot and ankle examination was normal, as was examination of her other major joints. A careful neurologic examination of the upper and lower extremities revealed no evidence of peripheral or entrapment neuropathy, and the deep tendon reflexes were normal.

Key Clinical Points—What's Important and What's Not

THE HISTORY

- A distant history of acute trauma to the right ankle
- No fever or chills
- Gradual onset of right anterior foot pain over the last several weeks with exacerbation of pain with foot use
- Difficulty working as dance instructor due to increased foot pain

THE PHYSICAL EXAMINATION

- Patient is afebrile
- Normal visual inspection of ankle and foot
- Palpation of dorsum of the right ankle and foot reveals diffuse tenderness
- No evidence of infection
- Pain reproduced with dorsiflexion and plantar flexion of the right ankle and foot

OTHER FINDINGS OF NOTE

- Normal blood pressure
- Normal HEENT examination

- Normal cardiovascular examination
- Normal pulmonary examination
- Normal abdominal examination
- No peripheral edema
- Normal upper extremity neurologic examination, motor and sensory examination
- Examinations of joints other than the right ankle were normal

 ## What Tests Would You Like to Order?

The following tests were ordered:
- Plain radiographs of the right ankle and foot

TEST RESULTS

The plain radiographs of the right foot revealed significant joint space narrowing and cartilage loss of the tarsal joints consistent with severe osteoarthritis (Fig. 2.1).

 ## Clinical Correlation—Putting It All Together

What is the diagnosis?
- Osteoarthritis of the right midtarsal joint

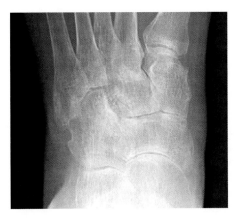

Fig. 2.1 Anteroposterior view of the midfoot demonstrating uniform cartilage loss between all the tarsal bones. (From Brower AC, Flemming DJ, eds. Rheumatoid arthritis. In: *Arthritis in Black and White*. ed. 3. Philadelphia: Saunders; 2012;170–199.)

The Science Behind the Diagnosis

ANATOMY OF THE MIDTARSAL JOINT

Each joint of the midtarsus has its own capsule (Fig. 2.2). The articular surface of each of these joints is covered with hyaline cartilage, which is susceptible to arthritis (Fig. 2.3). The midtarsal joint capsules are lined with a synovial membrane that attaches to the articular cartilage and allows the gliding motion of the joints. Various ligaments provide the majority of strength to the midtarsal joints. The muscles of the midtarsal joint and their attaching tendons are susceptible to trauma and to wear and tear from overuse and misuse.

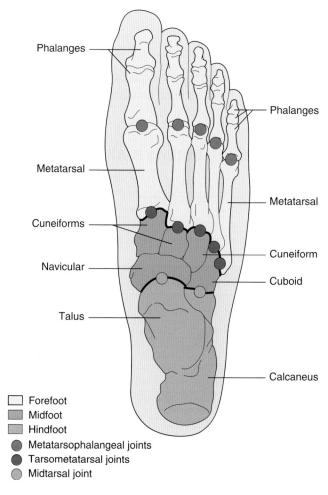

Fig. 2.2 The bones of the foot (superior view). (From Hochberg H, Silman AJ, Smolen JS, et al., eds. *Rheumatology*. ed. 3. Edinburgh, UK: Mosby, 2003.)

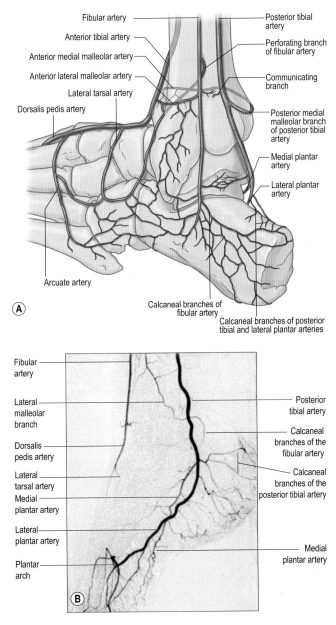

Fig. 2.3 (A) The bones of the foot. Each joint of the midtarsus has its own capsule. The articular surface of each of these joints is covered with hyaline cartilage, which is susceptible to arthritis. Also note the arterial supply which is susceptible to compromise by trauma, tumor, thrombus, and clot. (B) Arteriogram of the distal ankle and foot. (From Standring S. *Gray's Anatomy: The Anatomic Basis of Clinical Practice.* ed. 42. Elsevier; 2021 [Fig. 79-9 A].)

THE CLINICAL SYNDROME

Arthritis of the midtarsal joints is a common condition. The midtarsal joints are susceptible to the development of arthritis from various conditions that can damage the joint cartilage. Osteoarthritis is the most common form of arthritis that results in midtarsal joint pain; rheumatoid arthritis and posttraumatic arthritis are also frequent causes of midtarsal pain. Less common causes include the collagen vascular diseases, infection, and Lyme disease. Acute infectious arthritis is usually accompanied by significant systemic symptoms, including fever and malaise, and should be easily recognized; it is treated with culture and antibiotics rather than injection therapy. Charcot midtarsal joints may occur from a variety of peripheral neuropathies (Fig. 2.4). Collagen vascular disease generally manifests as polyarthropathy rather than as monoarthropathy limited to the midtarsal joint, although midtarsal pain secondary to collagen vascular disease responds exceedingly well to the treatment modalities described here.

Most patients present with pain localized to the dorsum of the foot. Activity, especially that involving inversion and adduction of the midtarsal joint, worsens the pain (Fig. 2.5), whereas rest and heat provide some relief. The pain is constant and is characterized as aching; it may interfere with sleep. Some patients complain of a grating or popping sensation with use of the joints, and crepitus may be present on physical examination. In addition to pain, patients with arthritis of the midtarsal joint often experience a gradual decrease in functional ability because of reduced midtarsal range of motion that makes simple everyday tasks, such as walking and climbing stairs, quite difficult.

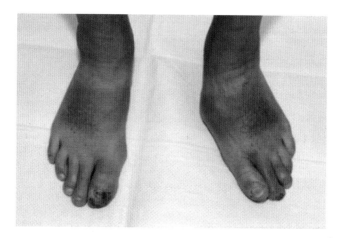

Fig. 2.4 Charcot neuroarthropathy of the midtarsal joint manifests as pain in the dorsum of the foot that is made worse with inversion and adduction of the affected joint. (From Young N, Neiderer K, Martin B, et al. HIV neuropathy induced Charcot neuroarthropathy: a case discussion. *Foot (Edinb).* 2012;22(3):112—116.)

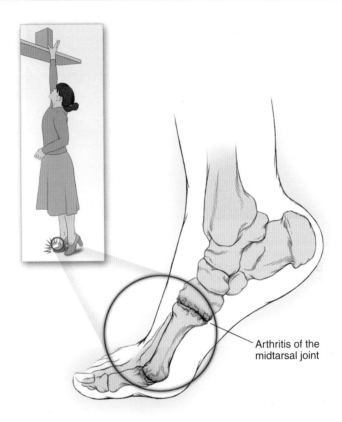

Arthritis of the
midtarsal joint

Fig. 2.5 The midtarsal joints are susceptible to the development of arthritis from various conditions that can damage the joint cartilage. (From Waldman S. *Atlas of Common Pain Syndromes*. ed. 4. Philadelphia: Elsevier; 2019 [Fig. 122-1].)

TESTING

Plain radiographs and ultrasound imaging are indicated for all patients who present with midtarsal pain (Fig. 2.6; see Fig. 2.1). Magnetic resonance imaging (MRI) of the midtarsal joint is indicated if aseptic necrosis, inflammatory arthritis, an occult mass, or a tumor is suspected as well as to confirm the diagnosis (Figs. 2.7, 2.8, and 2.9). Computed tomography scanning may be useful in further defining the pathology responsible for the patient's pain and functional disability. Based on the patient's clinical presentation, additional testing may be warranted, including a complete blood count, comprehensive metabolic profile, erythrocyte sedimentation rate, and antinuclear antibody testing.

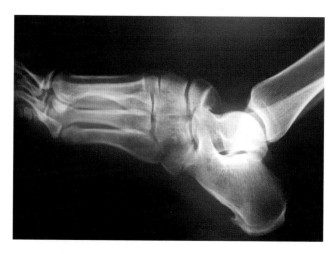

Fig. 2.6 Dislocation of the midtarsal joint. Oblique radiograph of the right foot showing dislocation of the talonavicular joint and subluxation of the calcaneocuboid joint. (From Puthezhath K, Veluthedath R, Kumaran CM, et al. Acute isolated dorsal midtarsal (Chopart's) dislocation: a case report. *J Foot Ankle Surg.* 2009;48(4):462−465 [Fig. 1]. ISSN 1067-2516, https://doi.org/10.1053/j.jfas.2009.01.016, http://www.sciencedirect.com/science/article/pii/S1067251609001082.)

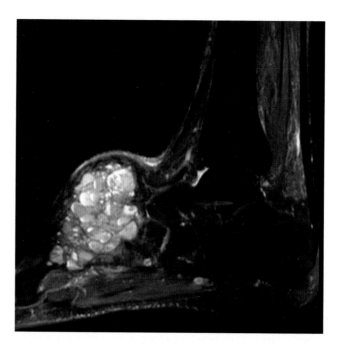

Fig. 2.7 Sagittal magnetic resonance imaging of the left foot. Aneurysmatic bone cyst originating from the first cuneiform resulting in a shoe conflict in a 25-year-old male patient. Before admission to our clinic, the tumorous mass was hidden in open sneakers and under wide jeans. (From Toepfer A. Tumors of the foot and ankle—a review of the principles of diagnostics and treatment. *Fuß & Sprunggelenk.* 2017;15 (2):82−96 [Fig. 4]. ISSN 1619-9987, https://doi.org/10.1016/j.fuspru.2017.03.004, http://www.science direct.com/science/article/pii/S1619998717300399.)

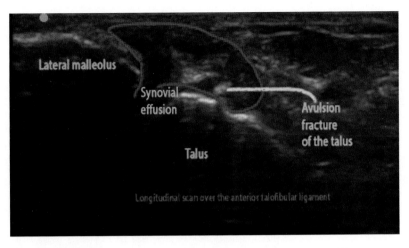

Fig. 2.8 Longitudinal ultrasound image demonstrating an avulsion fracture of the talus in a patient who suffered a severe inversion injury to the anterior talofibular ligament.

DIFFERENTIAL DIAGNOSIS

Primary disorders of the foot, including gout and occult fractures, may mimic the pain and disability of arthritis of the midtarsal joint. Bursitis and plantar fasciitis of the foot, as well as entrapment neuropathies such as tarsal tunnel syndrome, may also confuse the diagnosis; these conditions may coexist with arthritis of the midtarsal joint. Primary and metastatic tumors of the foot may also manifest in a manner similar to arthritis of the midtarsal joint.

TREATMENT

Initial treatment of the pain and functional disability associated with arthritis of the midtarsal joint includes a combination of nonsteroidal anti-inflammatory drugs or cyclooxygenase-2 inhibitors and physical therapy. The local application of heat and cold may also be beneficial. Avoidance of repetitive activities that aggravate the patient's symptoms, as well as short-term immobilization of the midtarsal joint, may provide relief. For patients who do not respond to these treatment modalities, intraarticular injection of local anesthetic and steroid is a reasonable next step (Fig. 2.10). Physical modalities, including local heat and gentle range-of-motion exercises, should be introduced several days after the patient undergoes injection. Vigorous exercises should be avoided because they will exacerbate the patient's symptoms.

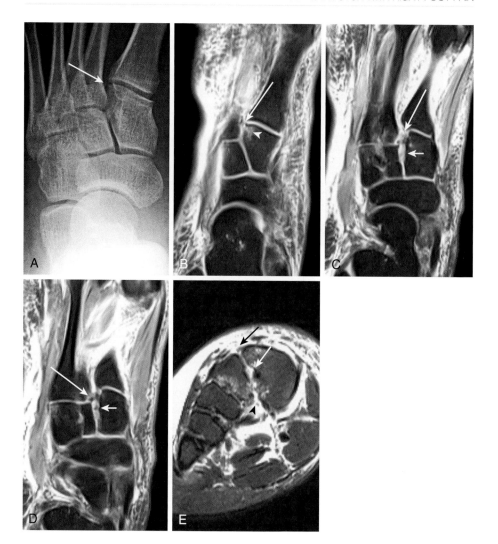

Fig. 2.9 Midfoot sprain suspected on radiographs and confirmed on magnetic resonance imaging (MRI). A 25-year-old woman injured her foot while running and twisting. Radiographs initially were interpreted as normal, and the patient was told to bear weight as tolerated. Radiographs at the author's institution were considered suspicious but not diagnostic for midfoot sprain, and MRI was performed. Fluoroscopy under anesthesia confirmed the MRI diagnosis of Lisfranc ligament complex rupture and instability of the first through third tarsometatarsal joints. (A) Anteroposterior weight-bearing radiograph shows a tiny chip fracture *(arrow)* arising either from the medial cuneiform or the first metatarsal. (B) Axial T2-weighted fat-saturated MRI obtained through the dorsum of foot shows a ruptured dorsal Lisfranc ligament *(arrow)* and bone marrow edema in the medial cuneiform *(arrowhead)*. (C) Axial T2-weighted fat-saturated MRI through midportion of the Lisfranc joint shows midsubstance rupture of the interosseous Lisfranc ligament *(long arrow)*. The first interosseous intercuneiform ligament *(short arrow)* is ruptured also. (D) Axial T2-weighted fat-saturated MRI through the plantar aspect of the Lisfranc joint shows small avulsion fragment from second metatarsal base *(long arrow)* that is not visible on radiographs. The first plantar intercuneiform ligament *(short arrow)* also is ruptured. (E) Coronal T2-weighted fat-saturated MRI through the Lisfranc joint demonstrates disruption of the dorsal Lisfranc ligament *(black arrow)*, the interosseous Lisfranc ligament *(white arrow)*, and the plantar Lisfranc ligament *(black arrowhead)*. (From Crim J. MR imaging evaluation of subtle Lisfranc injuries: the midfoot sprain. *Magn Res Imaging Clin North Am.* 2008;16:19—27.)

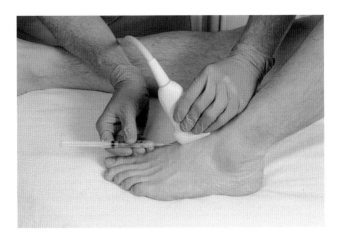

Fig. 2.10   Correct in-plane needle placement for ultrasound-guided talonavicular joint injection.

HIGH-YIELD TAKEAWAYS

- The patient is afebrile, making an acute infectious etiology (e.g., septic arthritis) unlikely.
- The patient's symptomatology is not the result of acute trauma but more likely the result of repetitive microtrauma that has damaged the joint over time.
- The patient's pain is diffuse rather than highly localized, as would be the case with a pathologic process such as Achilles tendinitis.
- The patient's symptoms are unilateral and involve only one joint, which is more suggestive of a local process than a systemic polyarthropathy.
- Plain radiographs will provide high-yield information regarding the bony contents of the joint, but ultrasound imaging and MRI will be more useful in identifying soft tissue pathology.

Suggested Readings

Alcaraz MJ, Megías J, García-Arnandis I, et al. New molecular targets for the treatment of osteoarthritis. *Biochem Pharmacol.* 2010;80(1):13—21.

Repetto I, Biti B, Cerruti P, et al. Conservative treatment of ankle osteoarthritis: can platelet-rich plasma effectively postpone surgery? *J Foot Ankle Surg.* 2017;56(2): 362—365.

Robinson AHN, Keith T. Osteoarthritis of the ankle. *Orthop Trauma.* 2016;30(1):59—67.

Waldman SD. Arthritis and other abnormalities of the ankle joint. In: *Waldman's Comprehensive Atlas of Diagnostic Ultrasound of Painful Conditions.* Philadelphia: Wolters Kluwer; 2016:875—882.

Waldman SD. Arthritis and other abnormalities of the talonavicular joint. In: *Waldman's Comprehensive Atlas of Diagnostic Ultrasound of Painful Conditions*. ed. 2. Philadelphia: Wolters Kluwer; 2016:889—896.

Waldman SD. Arthritis of the midtarsal joints. In: *Atlas of Common Pain Syndromes*. ed. 4. Philadelphia: Elsevier; 2019:484—486.

Waldman SD. Functional anatomy of the ankle and foot. In: *Pain Review*. ed. 2. Philadelphia: Elsevier; 2017:149—150.

Waldman SD. Intra-articular injection of the midtarsal joints. In: *Atlas of Pain Management Injection Techniques*. ed. 4. Philadelphia: Elsevier; 2017:593—595.

Waldman SD. Midtarsal joint pain. In: *Atlas of Uncommon Pain Syndromes*. ed. 4. Philadelphia: Elsevier; 2021:425—427.

Waldman SD. Ultrasound-guided intra-articular injection of the talonavicular joint. In: *Waldman's Comprehensive Atlas of Ultrasound Guided Pain Management Injection Techniques*. ed. 2. Philadelphia: Wolters Kluwer; 2020:1153—1157.

Waldman SD, Campbell RSD. Anatomy: special imaging considerations of the ankle and foot. In: *Imaging of Pain*. ed. 1. Philadelphia: Saunders; 2011:417—420.

Anna Coyle

A 24-Year-Old Dental Hygienist With Severe Medial Ankle Pain

- Learn the common causes of ankle pain.
- Develop an understanding of the unique anatomy of the ankle joint.
- Develop an understanding of the ligaments of the ankle.
- Develop an understanding of the causes of medial ankle pain.
- Develop an understanding of the differential diagnosis of deltoid ligament strain.
- Learn the clinical presentation of deltoid ligament strain.
- Learn how to examine the ankle and associated ligaments.
- Learn how to use physical examination to identify deltoid ligament strain.
- Develop an understanding of the treatment options for deltoid ligament strain.

Anna Coyle

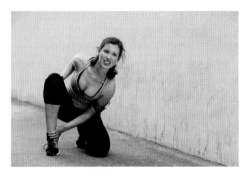

Anna Coyle is a 24-year-old dental hygienist with the chief complaint of, "I think I broke my ankle." Anna stated that about 2 weeks ago, she was running a half marathon and stepped into a pothole and twisted her ankle. She tried to finish the marathon, but the pain was just too bad. By the time she limped back to her car, her ankle was swollen and black and blue. She made it home and immediately iced and elevated the ankle. Over the past 10 days, the bruising and swelling have improved, but Anna states that the inside of her right ankle continues to hurt. Running has been out of the question, and the ankle pain has really been "messing with my running." I asked Anna if she ever had anything like this before, and she said, "I have had the usual aches and pains that you expect if you run marathons. Once I had what the shoe guy said was metatarsalgia when I didn't replace my running shoes. I learned my lesson that time. It's just hard to throw out expensive shoes! My ankle was fine until I stepped into that pothole. I twisted my ankle outward, and it felt like something on the inside of my ankle tore. It's been bothering me ever since."

I asked Anna what made the pain worse, and she said that any walking, weight bearing, walking on uneven surfaces, and putting on her jogging shoes all made the pain much worse. I asked her what made it better, and she said that she thought Advil helped, but it was upsetting her stomach. She noted that icing the ankle felt good, but the pain came back as soon as she took the ice off. I asked Anna about any other antecedent ankle trauma, and she said, "Not that I can recall."

I asked Anna to use one finger to point at the spot where it hurt the most. She pointed to her right medial ankle just below the medial malleolus.

On physical examination, Anna was afebrile. Her respirations were 16, and her pulse was 64 and regular. Her blood pressure was 126/80. Anna's head, eyes, ears, nose, throat (HEENT) exam was normal, as was her cardiopulmonary examination. Her thyroid was normal. Her abdominal examination revealed no abnormal mass or organomegaly. There was no costovertebral angle (CVA) tenderness. There was no peripheral edema. Her low back examination revealed some tenderness to deep palpation of the paraspinous musculature. Visual inspection of the right medial ankle revealed resolving ecchymosis, but the area appeared a little swollen. The area over the medial ankle felt a little warm but did not appear to be infected. The right medial ankle felt boggy on palpation. There was marked tenderness to palpation over the deltoid ligament, with the palpation of the area reproducing Anna's pain. Range of motion of the ankle joint, especially active resisted eversion and plantar flexion of the ankle joint, caused Anna to wince in pain. The left ankle examination was normal, as was examination of her major joints. The eversion test for deltoid ligament injury was markedly positive on the right, as was the rotary drawer test (Figs. 3.1 and 3.2). A careful neurologic examination of the upper and lower extremities revealed no evidence of peripheral or entrapment neuropathy, and the deep tendon reflexes were normal. I asked Anna to walk down the hall, where I noted an antalgic gait was present.

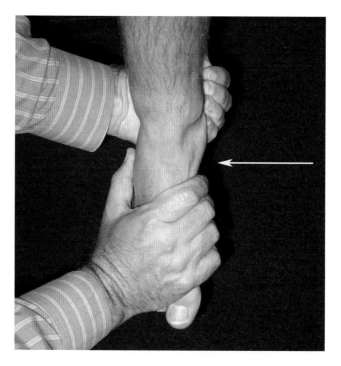

Fig. 3.1 Eversion test for deltoid ligament insufficiency. (From Waldman SD. *Physical Diagnosis of Pain: An Atlas of Signs and Symptoms*. Philadelphia: Saunders; 2006:369.)

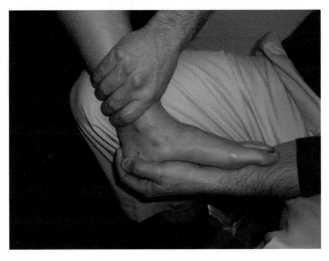

Fig. 3.2 Clinical image of rotatory drawer testing for medial ankle instability. (From Beals TC, Crim J, Nickisch F. Deltoid ligament injuries in athletes: techniques of repair and reconstruction. *Oper Techn Sport Med.* 2010;18(1):11−17 [Fig. 4]. ISSN 1060−1872, https://doi.org/10.1053/j.otsm.2009.10.001, http://www.sciencedirect.com/science/article/pii/S1060187209001233.)

Key Clinical Points—What's Important and What's Not

THE HISTORY

- Onset of right ankle pain following a jogging injury to the right ankle
- Pain localized to the area of the right deltoid ligament
- Pain made worse by walking, going down stairs, and walking on uneven surfaces
- No other specific traumatic events to the ankles
- No fever or chills
- Unable to jog due to persistent right ankle pain

THE PHYSICAL EXAMINATION

- Patient is afebrile
- Point tenderness to palpation of the area over the deltoid ligament
- Palpation of right ankle reveals warmth to touch
- Right medial ankle is swollen, with bogginess over the deltoid ligament
- No evidence of infection
- Pain on range of motion, especially active resisted eversion and plantar flexion of the affected right ankle
- Positive eversion test for deltoid ligament injury (see Fig. 3.1)

- Positive rotary drawer test for deltoid ligament injury (see Fig. 3.2)
- Antalgic gait is present

OTHER FINDINGS OF NOTE

- Normal HEENT examination
- Normal cardiovascular examination
- Normal pulmonary examination
- Normal abdominal examination
- No peripheral edema
- Normal upper and lower extremity neurologic examination, motor and sensory examination
- Examinations of joints other than the right ankle were normal

 ## What Tests Would You Like to Order?

The following tests were ordered:
- Plain radiographs of the right ankle
- Ultrasound of the right ankle

TEST RESULTS

The plain radiographs of the right ankle revealed mild soft tissue swelling over the medial ankle and a small medial malleolar avulsion fracture (Fig. 3.3).

Ultrasound examination of the right ankle revealed neovascularization of the deltoid ligament on color Doppler (Fig. 3.4).

 ## Clinical Correlation—Putting It All Together

What is the diagnosis?
- Deltoid ligament strain

The Science Behind the Diagnosis

ANATOMY

The ankle is a hinge-type articulation among the distal tibia, the two malleoli, and the talus. The articular surface is covered with hyaline cartilage, which is susceptible to arthritis. The joint is surrounded by a dense capsule that helps strengthen the ankle. The joint capsule is lined with a synovial membrane that attaches to the articular cartilage. The ankle joint is innervated by the deep peroneal and tibial nerves.

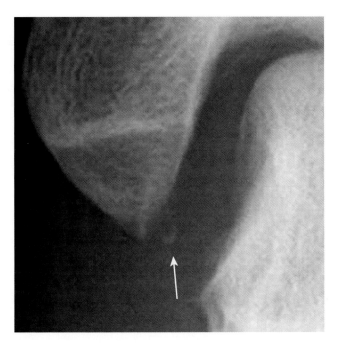

Fig. 3.3 Radiographic example of small avulsion of deltoid ligament with widened medial clear space. Arrow denotes the small bony avulsion. (Courtesy Thomas O. Clanton, MD.)

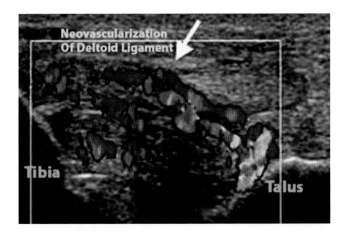

Fig. 3.4 Ultrasound examination of the right ankle revealed neovascularization of the deltoid ligament on color Doppler.

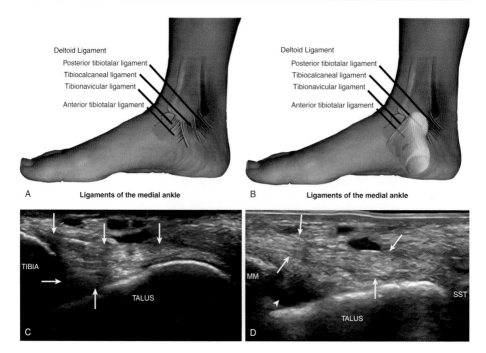

Fig. 3.5 Ligaments of the medial ankle. (A) Normal deltoid ligament. Note the navicular, talar, and calcaneal components. (B) Positioning of the transducer for the anterior tibiotalar portion of the ligament. (C) Normal anterior tibiotalar deltoid ligament *(arrows)*. Note the triangular echogenic appearance of the ligament. (D) Normal tibiocalcaneal portion of the deltoid ligament. Note the hyperechoic tibiocalcaneal ligament running from the medial malleolus to the sustentaculum tali *(arrows)*. Note also the small effusion in the ankle *(arrowhead)*. *MM*, Medial malleolus; *SST*, sustentaculum tali. (From Craig JG: Ultrasound of ligaments and bone. *Ultrasound Clin.* 2007;2:617–637.)

The major ligaments of the ankle joint include the deltoid, anterior talofibular, calcaneofibular, and posterior talofibular ligaments, which provide the majority of strength to the ankle joint (Fig. 3.5). The deltoid ligament is exceptionally strong and is not as subject to strain as the anterior talofibular ligament, and it has two layers (Fig. 3.6). Both layers attach above to the medial malleolus (Fig. 3.7). A deep layer attaches below to the medial body of the talus, with the superficial fibers attaching to the medial talus, the sustentaculum tali of the calcaneus, and the navicular tuberosity (Fig. 3.8).

CLINICAL SYNDROME

The deltoid ligament is exceptionally strong and is not as easily strained as is the anterior talofibular ligament. However, the deltoid ligament is susceptible to strain from acute injury resulting from sudden overeversion of the ankle or repetitive microtrauma to the ligament from overuse or misuse, such as

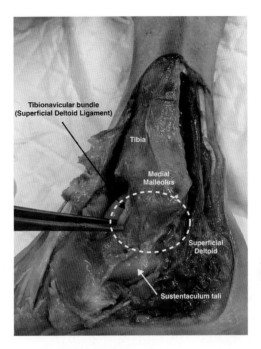

Fig. 3.6 Antero-medial view of the ankle after tibialis posterior, flexor hallucis longus and flexor digitorum longus tendons excision; the forceps point to the tibionavicular bundle. (From Guerra-Pinto, F, Fabian, A, Mota, T, et al. The tibiocalcaneal bundle of the deltoid ligament – prevalence and variations. *Foot and Ankle Surgery*. 2021;27(2):138–142 [Fig. 2].)

long-distance running on soft or uneven surfaces (Fig. 3.9). The deltoid ligament has two layers, both of which attach to the medial malleolus above it (Fig. 3.10). The deep layer attaches below to the medial body of the talus, and the superficial fibers attach to the medial talus, the sustentaculum tali of the calcaneus, and the navicular tuberosity.

SIGNS AND SYMPTOMS

Patients with deltoid ligament strain complain of pain just below the medial malleolus. Plantar flexion and eversion of the ankle joint exacerbate the pain. Often, patients with injury to the deltoid ligament note a pop, followed by significant swelling and the inability to walk (Fig. 3.11). On physical examination, patients have point tenderness over the medial malleolus. With acute trauma, ecchymosis over the ligament may be noted. Patients with deltoid ligament strain have a positive result of the eversion test, which is performed by passively everting and plantar flexing the affected ankle joint (see Fig. 3.1). Patients with deltoid ligament strain will also have a positive rotary drawer test, which is performed by cupping the heel of the affected foot and bringing the heel forward while at the same time

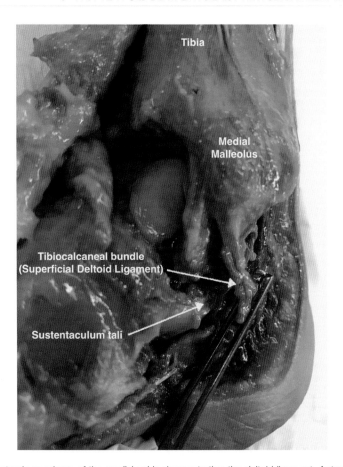

Fig. 3.7 Anatomic specimen of the medial ankle demonstrating the deltoid ligament. Anteromedial view of the ankle; the forceps show the tibiocalcaneal bundle of the superficial deltoid liagament after cutting it from the sustentaculum tali. The tibionavicular and tibiospring ligaments were cut from their distal insertion. (From Guerra-Pinto F, Fabian A, Mota T, et al. The tibiocalcaneal bundle of the deltoid ligament—prevalence and variations. *Foot Ankle Surg.* 2021;27(2):138–142. https://doi.org/10.1016/j.fas.2020.03.014. Epub 2020 Apr 28. PMID: 32381451.)

stabilizing the tibia with the opposite hand. In the case of superficial deltoid insufficiency, enhanced external rotation of the talus is observed when compared with the contralateral side (see Fig. 3.2). Coexistent bursitis and arthritis of the ankle and subtalar joint may also be present and may confuse the clinical picture.

TESTING

Plain radiographs are indicated for all patients who present with ankle pain (Fig. 3.12). Magnetic resonance imaging (MRI) and ultrasound imaging of the

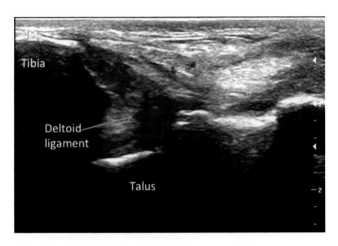

Fig. 3.8   Longitudinal ultrasound image demonstrating the triangular-shaped deltoid ligament.

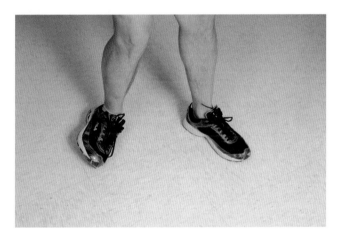

Fig. 3.9   The deltoid ligament is frequently injured by eversion injuries that occur when tripping while wearing high heels, landing hard on uneven surfaces, and during dancing, soccer, and American football.

ankle are indicated if disruption of the deltoid ligament, joint instability, an occult mass, or a tumor is suspected (Figs. 3.13 and 3.14). Bone scan should be performed if occult fracture is suspected. Based on the patient's clinical presentation, additional testing may be warranted, including a complete blood count, erythrocyte sedimentation rate, and antinuclear antibody testing.

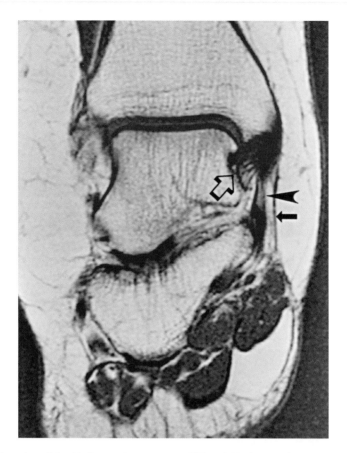

Fig. 3.10 Normal medial ankle ligaments on a coronal T1-weighted magnetic resonance image. The two layers of the deltoid (medial) ligament are seen. The deep tibiotalar ligament is striated *(open arrow)*. The more superficial tibiocalcaneal ligament *(arrowhead)* may have vertical striations as well. The thin, vertical, low-signal structure superficial to the tibiocalcaneal ligament is the flexor retinaculum *(solid arrow)*. (From Kaplan PA, Helms CA, Dussault R, et al. *Musculoskeletal MRI*. Philadelphia: Saunders; 2001:835.)

DIFFERENTIAL DIAGNOSIS

Avulsion fracture of the calcaneus, talus, medial malleolus, or base of the fifth metatarsal can mimic deltoid ligament pain. Bursitis, tendinitis, and gout of the midtarsal joints may coexist with deltoid ligament strain, thus confusing the diagnosis. Tarsal tunnel syndrome may occur after ankle trauma and further complicate the clinical picture (Box 3.1).

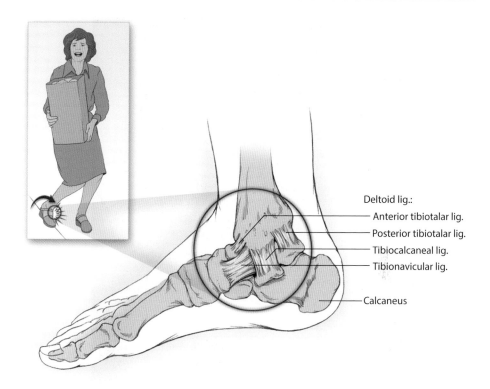

Deltoid lig.:
Anterior tibiotalar lig.
Posterior tibiotalar lig.
Tibiocalcaneal lig.
Tibionavicular lig.

Calcaneus

Fig. 3.11 With deltoid ligament strain, patients may notice a pop, followed by significant swelling. (From Waldman S. *Atlas of Common Pain Syndromes*. ed. 4. Philadelphia: Elsevier; 2019 [Fig. 123.2].)

TREATMENT

Initial treatment of the pain and functional disability associated with deltoid ligament strain includes a combination of nonsteroidal antiinflammatory drugs (NSAIDs) or cyclooxygenase-2 inhibitors and physical therapy. The local application of heat and cold may also be beneficial. Avoidance of repetitive activities that aggravate the patient's symptoms, as well as short-term immobilization of the ankle joint, may provide relief. For patients who do not respond to these treatment modalities, injection of the deltoid ligament with local anesthetic and steroid as both a diagnostic and therapeutic maneuver is a reasonable next step (Fig. 3.15). The injection of platelet-rich plasma and/or stem cells may reduce the pain and functional disability of deltoid ligament injuries. Physical modalities, including local heat and gentle range-of-motion exercises, should be introduced several days after the patient undergoes injection. Vigorous exercises should be avoided because they will exacerbate the patient's symptoms. Simple analgesics and NSAIDs can be used concurrently with this injection technique.

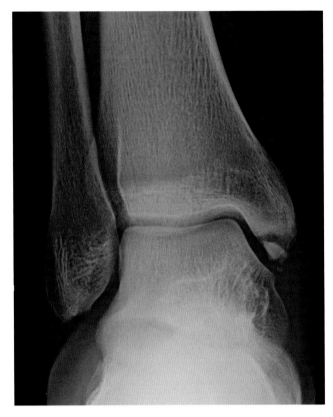

Fig. 3.12 Radiograph of larger medial malleolar avulsion injury in elite snowboarder. (Courtesy Thomas O. Clanton, MD.)

HIGH-YIELD TAKEAWAYS

- The patient is afebrile, making an acute infectious etiology (e.g., septic arthritis) unlikely.
- The patient's symptomatology is the result of acute trauma, and physical examination and testing should focus on the identification of ligamentous injury, acute arthritis, tendinitis, and bursitis.
- The patient has point tenderness over the deltoid ligament, which is highly suggestive of deltoid ligament strain.
- There is warmth and swelling of the area overlying the deltoid ligament, suggestive of an inflammatory process.

(Continued)

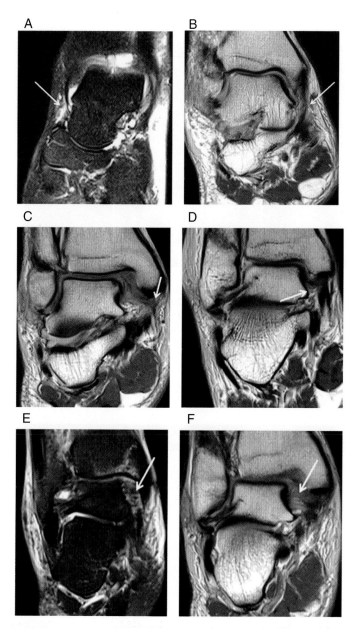

Fig. 3.13 Magnetic resonance image grading of deltoid ligament injury. (A) Grade I injury (TN, TS) of the anterior deltoid ligament (16-year-old boy with SER IV injury). (B) Grade II injury (TC, TS) of the anterior deltoid ligament (61-year-old woman with SER IV injury). (C) Grade III injury (TC, TS) of the anterior deltoid ligament (43-year-old man with SER IV injury). (D) Grade I injury (PTT) of the posterior deltoid ligament (18-year-old man with SER IV injury). (E) Grade II injury (PTT) of the posterior deltoid ligament (16-year-old boy with SER IV injury). (F) Grade III injury (PTT) of the posterior deltoid ligament (43-year-old man with SER IV injury). PTT, Posterior tibiotalar ligament; SER, supination external rotation; TC, tibiocalcaneal ligament; TN, tibionavicular ligament; TS, tibiospring ligament. (From Lee TH, Jang KS, Choi GW, et al. The contribution of anterior deltoid ligament to ankle stability in isolated lateral malleolar fractures. *Injury.* 2016;47(7):1581–1585 [Fig. 3]. ISSN 0020-1383, https://doi.org/10.1016/j.injury.2016.03.017, http://www.sciencedirect.com/science/article/pii/S0020138316300444.)

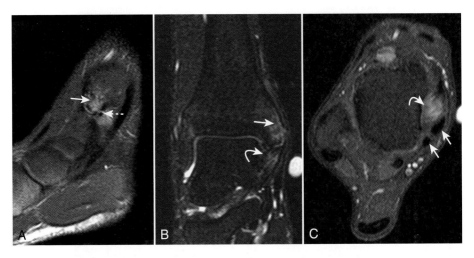

Fig. 3.14   Magnetic resonance imaging (MRI) of an ankle eversion injury. (A) Sagittal fat-suppressed T2-weighted (FST2W) MRI of an athlete with a subacute eversion ankle sprain. There is marrow edema in the tip of the medial malleolus *(white arrow)* and a possible small bony avulsion injury *(broken white arrow)*. (B) The coronal FST2W MRI also shows the marrow edema *(white arrow)*, and there is high signal intensity (SI) within the deltoid ligament *(curved white arrow)* as a result of partial tearing. (C) Consecutive axial FST2W MRIs more clearly demonstrate the deltoid ligament edema *(curved white arrow)* anterior to the flexor tendons *(white arrows)*. (From Waldman SD, Campbell RSD. *Imaging of Pain*. Philadelphia: Elsevier; 2011.)

BOX 3.1 ■ Differential Diagnosis of Ankle Sprain

- Avulsion fracture of the medial malleolus
- Tibial stress fracture
- Ostochondral injuries
- Os trigonum injury
- Talar fractures
- Spring ligament strain
- Calcaneal fractures
- Avulsion fractures of the calcaneus and cuboids
- Tendinitis
- Tarsal tunnel syndrome
- Arthritis
- Muscle tears

- The patient's symptoms are unilateral and involve only one joint, which is more suggestive of a local process than a systemic polyarthropathy.
- Plain radiographs will provide high-yield information regarding the bony contents of the joint and the identification of fractures or other bony abnormalities of the femur as well as calcification of the bursa and tendons, but ultrasound imaging and MRI will be more useful in identifying soft tissue pathology.

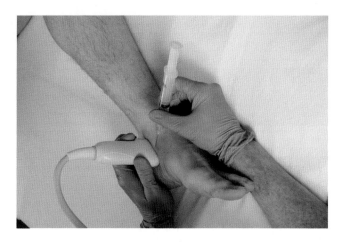

Fig. 3.15   Correct out-of-plane needle placement for ultrasound-guided deltoid ligament injection.

Suggested Readings

Alshalawi S, Galhoum AE, Alrashidi Y, et al. Medial ankle instability: the deltoid dilemma. *Foot Ankle Clin.* 2018;23(4):639–657.

Crim J. Medial-sided ankle pain: deltoid ligament and beyond. *Magn Res Imag Clin North Am.* 2017;25(1):63–77.

Waldman SD. Abnormalities of the deltoid ligament. In: *Waldman's Comprehensive Atlas of Ultrasound Diagnosis of Painful Conditions.* ed. 2. Philadelphia: Wolters Kluwer; 2016:905–910.

Waldman SD. Deltoid ligament strain. In: *Atlas of Common Pain Syndromes.* ed. 4. Philadelphia: Elsevier; 2019:487–491.

Waldman SD. Functional anatomy of the ankle and foot. In: *Pain Review.* ed. 2. Philadelphia: Saunders Elsevier; 2016:149–150.

Waldman SD. The deltoid ligament. In: *Pain Review.* ed. 2. Philadelphia: Saunders Elsevier; 2016:150–151.

Waldman SD, Campbell RSD. Deltoid ligament tear. In: *Imaging of Pain.* ed. 1. Philadelphia: Saunders Elsevier; 2010;439–442.

Scott English

A 32-Year-Old Truck Mechanic With Pain and Electric Shocklike Sensation Radiating Into the Dorsum of the Foot

Scott English

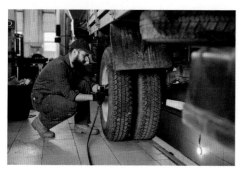

Scott English is a 32-year-old truck mechanic who has been my patient for the last several years. I last saw him for a subungual hematoma after he mashed his thumb with a hammer (Fig. 4.1). His chief complaint today is, "The top of my foot is going to sleep." Scott stated that over the past several months, in addition to the numbness, he began waking up at night with deep, aching right foot pain. "At first, I thought it was those damned steel-toed shoes that they make me wear. I think they make me wear them because if I get injured, they only have to pay worker's comp on a couple of toes getting chopped off by the steel rather than a bunch of crushed toes! In this state, a chopped off big toe isn't worth much. Anyway, I just got a new pair of steel-toed shoes, and at first I thought they would fit fine after I broke them in, but they are just a smidge tight across the top of my foot. I don't tie them very tight, but they still pinch the top of my foot. I wore them, so I can't take them back."

I asked Scott if he had experienced any other symptoms, and he replied, "Doc, it's funny that you asked because I noticed that when I wash between my toes, the duck web between my big toe and the next one is kind of numb. That's really crazy, isn't it? I am having a real hard time when I have to squat down to check a tire pressure or patch a tire. If I squat for too long, the top of my right foot gets these little electric shocks. It makes me want to scream. Not that it hurts that bad, it just really gets on your nerves, and I absolutely have to stand up. I have to be careful when the boss is around. He is always giving me the hairy eyeball." I asked Scott what he had tried to make it better, and he said that taking his shoes off was about the only thing that helped. Scott went on to say that he tried to use a heating pad on his foot when he got home from work, and it "seemed to make the pins and needles worse. Tylenol PM seemed to help some, at least with sleep. You know, I have to be really careful what I take because I never know when that jackass I work for is going to make me pee in a cup." I asked Scott about any fever, chills, or other constitutional symptoms such as weight loss or night sweats, and he shook his head no. He denied any antecedent foot trauma, but he again noted that most nights, the foot pain woke him.

I asked Scott to point with one finger to show me where it hurt the most. He pointed to the dorsum of the right foot. He went on to say that he could live with the numbness between the toes, "but the crazy way the top of my foot feels kind of scares me. I have to be able to squat if I want to keep my job." He then asked,

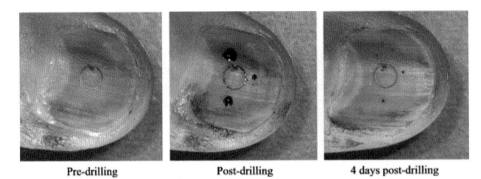

| Pre-drilling | Post-drilling | 4 days post-drilling |

Fig. 4.1 Subungual hematoma. Before and after hematoma evacuation. (From Salter SA, Ciocon DH, Gowrishankar TR, et al. Controlled nail trephination for subungual hematoma. *Am J Emerg Med.* 2006;24(7):875–877 [Fig. 3]. ISSN 0735-6757, https://doi.org/10.1016/j.ajem.2006.03.029, http://www.sciencedirect.com/science/article/pii/S0735675706001409.)

"Doc, do you think I can get the worker's comp or go on disability?" I said that I thought that would be a heavy lift, but that I would do everything I could to get him better.

On physical examination, Scott was afebrile. His respirations were 16, his pulse was 64 and regular, and his blood pressure was 110/68. Scott's head, eyes, ears, nose, throat (HEENT) exam was normal, as was his cardiopulmonary examination. His thyroid was normal. His abdominal examination revealed no abnormal mass or organomegaly. There was no costovertebral angle (CVA) tenderness. There was no peripheral edema. His low back examination was unremarkable. Visual inspection of the right foot was unremarkable. There was no ecchymosis, rubor, or color, and there was no obvious infection. There was a positive Tinel sign over the right deep peroneal nerve at the foot. There was weakness of the extensor digitorum brevis on the right. Examination of Scott's toes revealed no stigmata of osteoarthritis or rheumatoid arthritis. The left foot examination was normal. A careful neurologic examination of the lower extremities revealed decreased sensation in the distribution of the distal deep peroneal nerve (Fig. 4.2). Deep tendon reflexes were normal. Scott exhibited a positive Tinel sign over the deep peroneal nerve (Fig. 4.3).

Key Clinical Points—What's Important and What's Not

THE HISTORY

■ A history of the onset of right foot pain with associated paresthesias into the distribution of the deep peroneal nerve

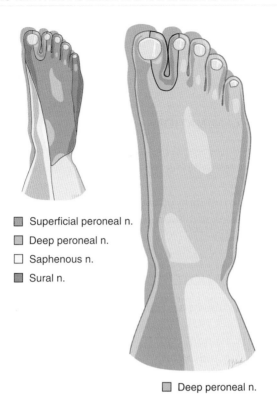

Superficial peroneal n.

Deep peroneal n.

Saphenous n.

Sural n.

Deep peroneal n.

Fig. 4.2 The sensory distribution of the deep peroneal nerve. (From Waldman S. *Atlas of Interventional Pain Management*. ed. 5. Philadelphia: Elsevier; 2021 [Fig. 152.4].)

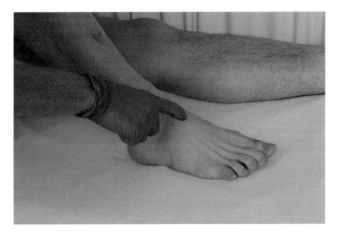

Fig. 4.3 A positive Tinel sign just medial to the dorsalis pedis pulse over the deep peroneal nerve as it passes beneath the fascia is usually present in patients suffering from anterior tarsal tunnel syndrome.

- Numbness of the web space between the big and second toe on the right
- Foot weakness
- No history of previous significant foot pain
- No fever or chills

THE PHYSICAL EXAMINATION

- Patient is afebrile
- Positive Tinel sign over the deep peroneal nerve at the dorsum of the right foot (see Fig. 4.3)
- Numbness in the distribution of the deep peroneal nerve (see Fig. 4.2)
- Weakness of the extensor digitorum brevis
- No evidence of infection

OTHER FINDINGS OF NOTE

- Normal HEENT examination
- Normal cardiovascular examination
- Normal pulmonary examination
- Normal abdominal examination
- No peripheral edema
- Normal left upper extremity neurologic examination, motor and sensory examination

 What Tests Would You Like to Order?

The following tests were ordered:
- Electromyography (EMG) and nerve conduction velocity testing of the right upper extremity
- Ultrasound of the right foot
- Magnetic resonance imaging (MRI) of the right foot

TEST RESULTS

EMG and nerve conduction velocity testing revealed slowing of deep peroneal nerve conduction across the ankle.

Ultrasound examination of the right foot revealed flattening and enlargement of the deep peroneal nerve as it passed beneath the superficial fascia (Fig. 4.4).

MRI scan of the right foot revealed osteoarthritis of the ankle and subtalar joint with a prominent osteophyte displacing the neurovascular bundle (Fig. 4.5).

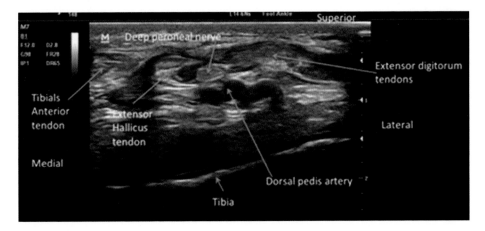

Fig. 4.4 Transverse ultrasound image demonstrating the tibial artery and vein and the deep peroneal nerve just above and lateral to the vein.

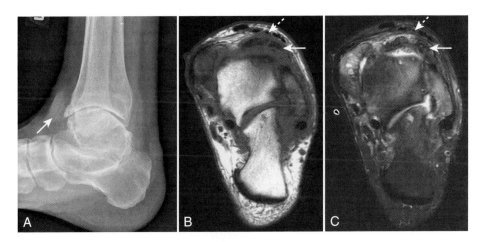

Fig. 4.5 Lateral radiograph of a patient with osteoarthritis of the ankle and subtalar joint. (A) There is prominent anterior osteophyte formation at the anterior aspect of the joint with associated soft tissue shadowing *(white arrow)*. The axial T1-weighted (T1W) (B) and T2W with fat suppression (C) magnetic resonance images show the anterior osteophytosis and associated synovitis *(white arrows)* impinging on the extensor tendons. The anterior tibial artery is displaced anteriorly *(broken white arrows)* between the extensor tendons. (From Waldman S, Campbell R. *Imaging of Pain.* ed. 1. Philadelphia: Saunders; 2011 [Fig. 164.2].)

Clinical Correlation—Putting It All Together

What is the diagnosis?

■ Anterior tarsal tunnel syndrome

The Science Behind the Diagnosis

ANATOMY

The common peroneal nerve is one of the two major continuations of the sciatic nerve, the other being the tibial nerve (Fig. 4.6). The common peroneal nerve, which is also known as the common fibular nerve, provides sensory innervation to the inferior portion of the knee joint and the posterior and lateral skin of the upper calf. The common peroneal nerve is derived from the posterior branches of the L4, L5, S1, and S2 nerve roots. The nerve splits from the sciatic nerve at the superior margin of the popliteal fossa and descends laterally behind the head of the fibula (Fig. 4.7). The common

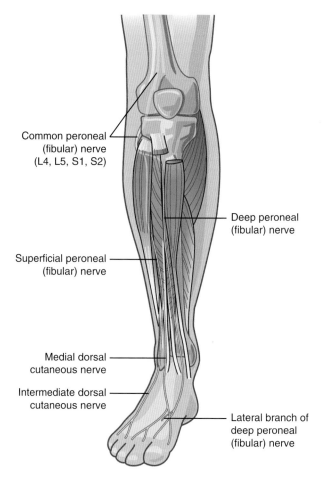

Fig. 4.6 Anatomy of the common peroneal nerve. (From Waldman S. *Atlas of Interventional Pain Management*. ed. 5. Philadelphia: Elsevier; 2021 [Fig. 150.5].)

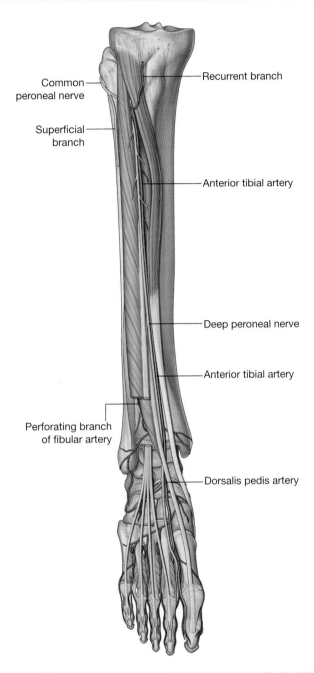

Fig. 4.7 The anatomy of the deep peroneal nerve. (Modified from Drake RL, Vogl W, Mitchell AWM. *Gray's Anatomy for Students*. Philadelphia: Churchill Livingstone; 2004.)

peroneal nerve is subject to compression at this point by such circumstances as improperly applied casts and tourniquets. The nerve is also subject to compression as it continues its lateral course, winding around the fibula through the fibular tunnel, which is made up of the posterior border of the tendinous insertion of the peroneus longus muscle and the fibula itself. Just distal to the fibular tunnel, the nerve divides into its two terminal branches, the superficial and the deep peroneal nerves (see Fig. 4.7). Each of these branches is subject to trauma and may be blocked individually as a diagnostic and therapeutic maneuver.

The deep branch of the peroneal nerve continues down the leg in conjunction with the tibial artery and vein to provide sensory innervation to the web space of the first and second toes and adjacent dorsum of the foot (see Fig. 4.2). Although this distribution of sensory fibers is small, this area is often the site of Morton neuroma surgery and thus is important to the regional anesthesiologist. The deep peroneal nerve provides motor innervation to all of the toe extensors and the anterior tibialis muscles. The deep peroneal nerve passes beneath the dense superficial fascia of the ankle, where it is subject to an entrapment syndrome known as the anterior tarsal tunnel syndrome (Fig. 4.8).

CLINICAL SYNDROME

Anterior tarsal tunnel syndrome is caused by compression of the deep peroneal nerve as it passes beneath the superficial fascia of the ankle (see Fig. 4.8). The most common cause of this compression is trauma to the dorsum of the foot. Severe, acute plantar flexion of the foot has been implicated in anterior tarsal tunnel syndrome, as has wearing tight shoes or squatting and bending forward, such as when planting flowers (Fig. 4.9). The syndrome has also been associated with hypertrophy of the extensor hallucis brevis muscle in dancers (Fig. 4.10). Anterior tarsal tunnel syndrome is much less common than posterior tarsal tunnel syndrome.

SIGNS AND SYMPTOMS

This entrapment neuropathy manifests primarily as pain, numbness, and paresthesias in the dorsum of the foot that radiate into the first dorsal web space; these symptoms may also radiate proximal to the entrapment, into the anterior ankle. No motor involvement occurs unless the distal lateral division of the deep peroneal nerve is affected. Nighttime foot pain analogous to that of carpal tunnel syndrome is often present. Patients may report that holding the foot in the everted position decreases the pain and paresthesias.

Physical findings include tenderness over the deep peroneal nerve at the dorsum of the foot. A positive Tinel sign just medial to the dorsalis pedis pulse over

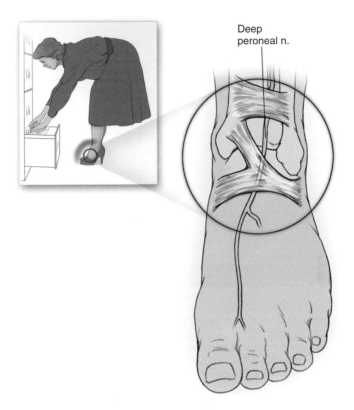

Deep
peroneal n.

Fig. 4.8 Anterior tarsal tunnel syndrome manifests as deep, aching pain in the dorsum of the foot, weakness of the extensor digitorum brevis, and numbness in the distribution of the deep peroneal nerve. (From Waldman S. *Atlas of Common Pain Syndromes*. ed. 4. Philadelphia: Elsevier; 2019 [Fig. 124.2].)

the deep peroneal nerve as it passes beneath the fascia is usually present (see Fig. 4.3). Active plantar flexion often reproduces the symptoms of anterior tarsal tunnel syndrome. Weakness of the extensor digitorum brevis may be present if the lateral branch of the deep peroneal nerve is affected.

TESTING

EMG can distinguish lumbar radiculopathy and diabetic polyneuropathy from anterior tarsal tunnel syndrome. Plain radiographs are indicated in all patients who present with foot or ankle pain to rule out occult bony disease (Fig. 4.11). MRI and ultrasound imaging of the ankle and foot are indicated if joint instability or a space-occupying lesion is suspected (Figs. 4.12 and 4.13). Based on the patient's clinical presentation, additional testing may be warranted, including a complete blood count, uric acid level, erythrocyte sedimentation rate, and

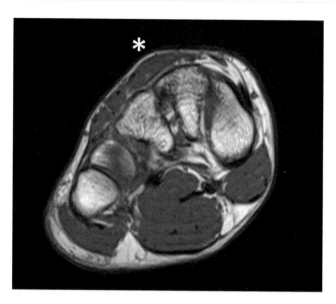

Fig. 4.9 T1-weighted magnetic resonance image coronal cut at midfoot showing hypertrophy of the extensor hallucis brevis (EHB) in a ballet dancer with anterior tarsal tunnel syndrome (* immediately dorsal to EHB). (From Tennant JN, Rungprai C, Phisitkul P. Bilateral anterior tarsal tunnel syndrome variant secondary to extensor hallucis brevis muscle hypertrophy in a ballet dancer: a case report. *Foot Ankle Surg.* 2014;20(4):e56–e58.)

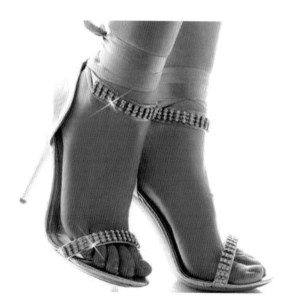

Fig. 4.10 Anterior tarsal tunnel syndrome can be caused by compression of the deep peroneal nerve by shoe straps or laces that are too tight. (From Waldman S. *Atlas of Interventional Pain Management.* ed. 5. Philadelphia: Elsevier; 2021 [Fig. 152.15].)

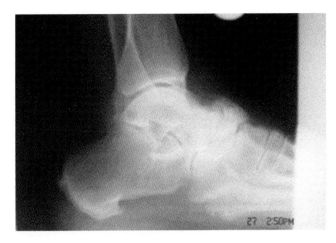

Fig. 4.11 Radiograph shows talar navicular exostosis, which causes compression to the deep peroneal nerve. (From DiDomenico LA, Masternick EB. Anterior tarsal tunnel syndrome. *Clin Podiatr Med Surg.* 2006;23(3):611–620 [Fig. 4]. ISSN 0891-8422, https://doi.org/10.1016/j.cpm.2006.04.007, http://www.sciencedirect.com/science/article/pii/S0891842206000243.)

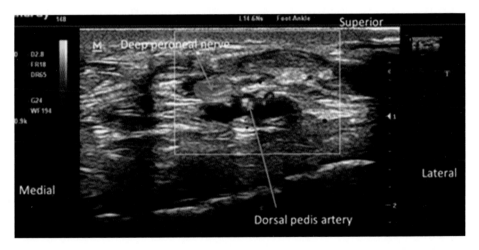

Fig. 4.12 Transverse color Doppler image demonstrating the popliteal vein and artery and the relationship of the vein to the deep peroneal nerve.

antinuclear antibody testing. The injection technique described later serves as both a diagnostic and a therapeutic maneuver.

DIFFERENTIAL DIAGNOSIS

Anterior tarsal tunnel syndrome is often misdiagnosed as arthritis of the ankle joint, lumbar radiculopathy, or diabetic polyneuropathy. Patients with arthritis

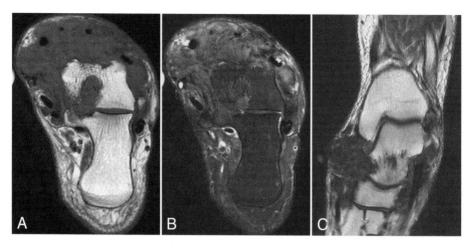

Fig. 4.13   Axial T1-weighted (A) and fat-suppressed t2-weighted (B) magnetic resonance images of a patient with ankle pain and paresthesia over the dorsal aspect of the foot. A mass of synovitis arising from the ankle joint surrounds the extensor tendons and the anterior neurovascular bundle. The synovium has intermediate signal intensity on both images and also on the coronal T2-weighted image (C). There is also bony erosion. These appearances are typical of pigmented villonodular synovitis. (From Waldman S, Campbell R. *Imaging of Pain*. Philadelphia: Saunders; 2011 [Fig. 164.3].)

of the ankle, however, have radiographic evidence of arthritis. Most patients suffering from lumbar radiculopathy have reflex, motor, and sensory changes associated with back pain, whereas patients with anterior tarsal tunnel syndrome have no reflex changes or motor deficits, and sensory changes are limited to the distribution of the distal deep peroneal nerve. However, lumbar radiculopathy and deep peroneal nerve entrapment may coexist as the double-crush syndrome. Diabetic polyneuropathy generally manifests as a symmetric sensory deficit involving the entire foot rather than a disorder limited to the distribution of the deep peroneal nerve. When anterior tarsal tunnel syndrome occurs in diabetic patients, diabetic polyneuropathy is usually also present.

TREATMENT

Mild cases of tarsal tunnel syndrome usually respond to conservative therapy; surgery should be reserved for severe cases. Initial treatment of tarsal tunnel syndrome consists of simple analgesics, nonsteroidal antiinflammatory drugs, or cyclooxygenase-2 inhibitors and splinting of the ankle. At a minimum, the splint should be worn at night, but wearing it for 24 hours a day is ideal. Avoidance of repetitive activities that may be responsible for the development of tarsal tunnel syndrome, such as prolonged squatting or wearing shoes that are too tight, can also ameliorate the symptoms. If patients fail to respond to these conservative measures, injection of the tarsal tunnel with local anesthetic and steroid is a

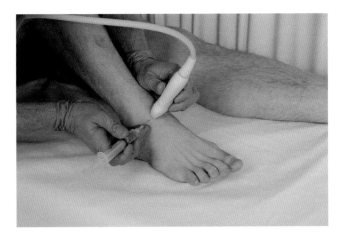

Fig. 4.14 Proper in-plane needle position for performing injection technique for anterior tarsal tunnel syndrome.

reasonable next step (Fig. 4.14). Surgical decompression of the deep peroneal nerve may be required in patients who fail to respond to more conservative measures (Fig. 4.15).

HIGH-YIELD TAKEAWAYS

- The patient is afebrile, making an acute infectious etiology unlikely.
- The patient's symptomatology is thought to be the result of compression of the deep peroneal nerve as it passes beneath the superficial fascia.
- Physical examination and testing should focus on identification of the various causes of deep peroneal nerve entrapment at the foot.
- The patient exhibits the neurologic and physical examination findings that are highly suggestive of deep peroneal nerve entrapment at the foot and anterior tarsal tunnel syndrome.
- The patient's symptoms are unilateral, which is more suggestive of a local process than a systemic inflammatory process such as polyneuropathy.
- Plain radiographs will provide high-yield information regarding the bony contents of the joint, but ultrasound imaging and MRI will be more useful in identifying soft tissue pathology that may be responsible for deep peroneal nerve compromise.
- EMG and nerve conduction velocity testing will help delineate the location and degree of nerve compromise if deep peroneal nerve compromise is suspected.

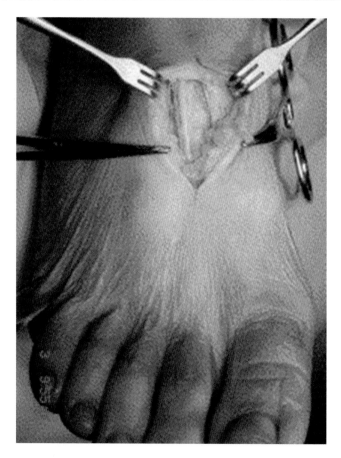

Fig. 4.15 Surgical decompression of the deep peroneal nerve may be required in patients who fail to respond to more conservative measures. An intraoperative view of the deep peroneal nerve after resection of the extensor hallucis brevis tendon. (From DiDomenico LA, Masternick EB. Anterior tarsal tunnel syndrome. *Clin Podiatr Med Surg.* 2006;23(3):611–620 [Fig. 5]. ISSN 0891-8422, https://doi.org/10.1016/j.cpm.2006.04.007, http://www.sciencedirect.com/science/article/pii/S0891842206000243.)

Suggested Readings

de Cesar Netto C, da Fonseca LF, Nascimento FS, et al. Diagnostic and therapeutic injections of the foot and ankle—an overview. *Foot Ankle Surg.* 2018;24(2):99–106.

DiDomenico LA, Masternick EB. Anterior tarsal tunnel syndrome. *Clin Podiatr Med Surg.* 2006;23(3):611–620.

Grant CRK, Raju PKBC. Lower limb nerve blocks. *Anaesth Intens Care Med.* 2016;17(4):182–186.

Kennedy JG, Baxter DE. Nerve disorders in dancers. *Clin Sports Med.* 2008;27(2):329–334.

Waldman SD. Anterior tarsal tunnel syndrome. In: *Atlas of Common Pain Syndromes.* ed. 4. Philadelphia: Elsevier; 2017:492–495.

Waldman SD. Anterior tarsal tunnel syndrome and other abnormalities of the deep peroneal nerve. In: *Waldman's Comprehensive Atlas of Ultrasound Diagnosis of Painful Conditions*. ed. 2. Philadelphia: Wolters Kluwer; 2016:940–951.

Waldman SD. Deep peroneal nerve block at the ankle. In: *Pain Review*. ed. 2. Philadelphia: Saunders; 2017:541–542.

Waldman SD, Campbell RSD. Anterior tarsal tunnel syndrome. In: *Imaging of Pain*. ed. 1. Philadelphia: Saunders; 2011:421–423.

Chip Anderson

A 36-Year-Old Maintenance Man With Numbness and Paresthesias in the Sole of the Foot

- Learn the common causes of foot pain.
- Learn the common causes of foot numbness.
- Develop an understanding of the unique relationship of the posterior tibial nerve to the flexor retinaculum and bones of the foot.
- Develop an understanding of the anatomy of the posterior tibial nerve.
- Develop an understanding of the causes of posterior tarsal tunnel syndrome.
- Develop an understanding of the differential diagnosis of posterior tarsal tunnel syndrome.
- Learn the clinical presentation of posterior tarsal tunnel syndrome.
- Learn how to examine the ankle and foot.
- Learn how to examine the posterior tibial nerve.
- Learn how to use physical examination to identify posterior tarsal tunnel syndrome.
- Develop an understanding of the treatment options for posterior tarsal tunnel syndrome.

Chip Andersen

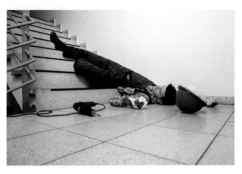

Chip Anderson is a 36-year-old maintenance man whom I have seen over the last several years. He came to the office today exclaiming, "Doctor, this time, I damn near got myself killed! I knew better, but I was in a hurry to get to lunch. I was hanging an emergency light on the stairs and didn't want to take time to go back to the shop and get the correct ladder. My gramps always said, 'haste makes waste'; now I know what he was talking about. The ladder slipped, and I tried to catch myself, but in the process I dislocated my ankle. Really stupid, huh? I definitely knew better. My ankle is getting better, but now I've got a numb foot and an irritating pins-and-needles sensation that shoots into the sole of my foot. I did my therapy just like I was supposed to, but it isn't getting better." I wouldn't say that Chip is accident prone, but he has certainly had his share of on-the-job injuries: smashed fingers, lacerations, corneal abrasions. I had also seen him for the usual upper respiratory tract infections.

I asked Chip if he had experienced any foot or toe weakness, and he replied, "Doc, it's funny that you asked. When I first got out of my cast, I thought it was just that my right foot was weak. And although I feel like I'm getting stronger every day, my foot feels like it's unstable. Kind of like it's squishy or flat—like I'm a cartoon character. It just doesn't feel right. The other thing is, the toes on the right don't seem to want to flex. After a day at work, especially if I'm on the stepladder a lot, I've been noticing that the bottom of my foot is really numb, and the pins-and-needles sensation is really aggravating." Chip was certainly a talker. "Let me ask you a few more questions, Chip, and examine you so we can figure out what's going on."

I asked Chip what he had tried to make it better. He said when he elevates his foot, it seems to make the pain better, and after about 30 to 40 minutes, the numbness gets a bit better. "The melatonin seemed to help some, at least with the sleep. I bet that foot wakes me up 10 times a night. I feel like I need to shake it to get it to wake up." I asked Chip about any fever, chills, or other constitutional symptoms such as weight loss or night sweats, and he shook his head no. He denied any other antecedent ankle or foot trauma. I took a look at copies of the x-rays that were taken on Chip's arrival at the emergency room, and I had to agree that he really did a number on his ankle. It was surpising that he was doing as well as he was, given the extent of the trauma (Fig. 5.1).

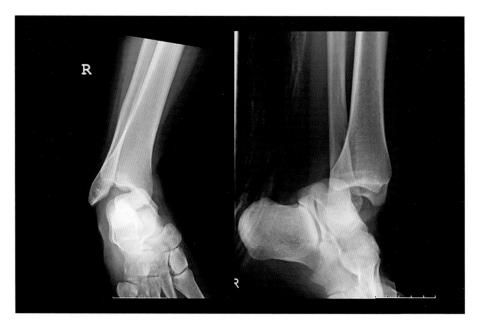

Fig. 5.1 X-ray of a posteromedial pure ankle dislocation. No fracture is noted. (From Wight L, Owen D, Goldbloom D, et al. Pure ankle dislocation: a systematic review of the literature and estimation of incidence. *Injury*. 2017;48(10):2027–2034 [Fig. 1]. ISSN 0020-1383, https://doi.org/10.1016/j.injury. 2017.08.011, http://www.sciencedirect.com/science/article/pii/S0020138317305259.)

I asked Chip to point with one finger to show me where it hurt the most. He pointed to an area just behind the medial malleolus and said that he felt like the pins-and-needles were coming from "right behind this bone right here." He then rubbed the bottom of his right foot and said that it was really numb.

On physical examination, Chip was afebrile. His respirations were 18, his pulse was 74 and regular, and his blood pressure was 120/72. Chip's head, eyes, ears, nose, throat (HEENT) exam was normal, as was his cardiopulmonary examination. His thyroid was normal. His abdominal examination revealed no abnormal mass or organomegaly. There was no costovertebral angle (CVA) tenderness. There was no peripheral edema. His low back examination was unremarkable. Visual inspection of the right ankle revealed a trace of edema, but there was no evidence of infection. The left foot and ankle were unremarkable. There was no rubor or calor. There was no obvious bony defect or tendinitis. There was a positive Tinel sign over the right posterior tibial nerve at the ankle (Fig. 5.2). There was weakness of the toe flexors and I noted some flattening of the arch of the foot, suggesting weakness of the lumbricals on the right. There was decreased sensation in the distribution of the posterior tibial nerve on the right. There was tenderness to palpation of the area behind the medial malleolus

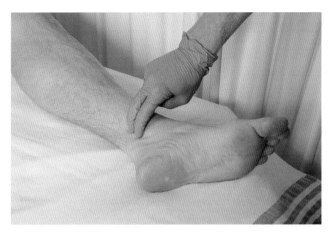

Fig. 5.2 Positive Tinel sign over the posterior tibial nerve is usually present in patients suffering from posterior tarsal tunnel syndrome.

on the right. A careful neurologic examination of the upper extremities was normal. I asked Chip to walk down the hall, where I saw that his gait was normal, which was pretty amazing, given the extent of his recent ankle injury.

Key Clinical Points—What's Important and What's Not

THE HISTORY

- History of ankle injury with a dislocation of the ankle
- History of onset of numbness of the sole of the right foot with associated paresthesias and numbness radiating into the distribution of the posterior tibial nerve
- No history of previous significant ankle or foot pain
- No fever or chills

THE PHYSICAL EXAMINATION

- Patient is afebrile
- Positive Tinel sign over the posterior tibial nerve at the ankle (see Fig. 5.2)
- Weakness of the toe flexors on the right
- Some flattening of the arch of the foot on the right, suggesting weakness of the lumbricals
- Numbness of the sole of the foot in the distribution of the posterior tibial nerve
- No evidence of infection

OTHER FINDINGS OF NOTE

- Normal HEENT examination
- Normal cardiovascular examination
- Normal pulmonary examination
- Normal abdominal examination
- No peripheral edema
- Normal upper extremity neurologic examination, motor and sensory examination

 ## What Tests Would You Like to Order?

The following tests were ordered:
- X-ray of the right ankle
- Electromyography (EMG) and nerve conduction velocity testing of the right lower extremity

TEST RESULTS

X-ray of the right ankle reveals good alignment of the tibiotalar joint without malleolar fractures (Fig. 5.3).

EMG and nerve conduction velocity testing revealed slowing of posterior tibial nerve conduction across the foot as well as denervation of the intrinsic muscles of the foot.

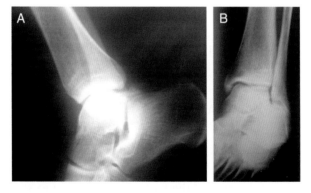

Fig. 5.3 Postreduction radiographs of (A) face and (B) profile showing good alignment of the tibiotalar joint without malleolar fractures. (From Lazarettos I, Brilakis E, Efstathopoulos N. Open ankle dislocation without associated malleolar fracture. *J Foot Ankle Surg.* 2013;52(4):508–512 [Fig. 2]. ISSN 1067-2516, https://doi.org/10.1053/j.jfas.2013.03.017, http://www.sciencedirect.com/science/article/pii/S106725161300118X.)

🗐 Clinical Correlation—Putting It All Together

What is the diagnosis?

■ Posterior tarsal tunnel syndrome

The Science Behind the Diagnosis

ANATOMY

The tibial nerve is one of two major continuations of the sciatic nerve, the other being the common peroneal nerve (Fig. 5.4). The tibial nerve provides sensory innervation to the posterior portion of the calf, the heel, and the medial plantar surface. The tibial nerve splits from the sciatic nerve at the superior margin of the popliteal fossa and descends in a slightly medial course through the popliteal fossa. The tibial nerve at the ankle lies just beneath the popliteal fascia and is readily

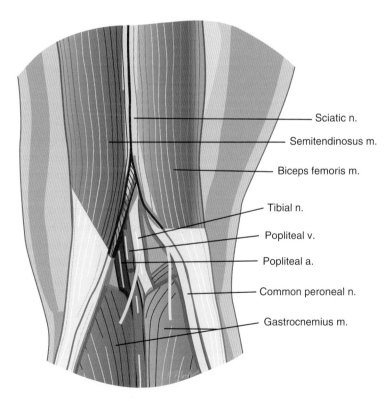

Fig. 5.4 The tibial nerve is one of two major continuations of the sciatic nerve, the other being the common peroneal nerve. (From Waldman S. *Atlas of Interventional Pain Management.* ed. 5. Philadelphia: Elsevier; 2021 [Fig. 147-2].)

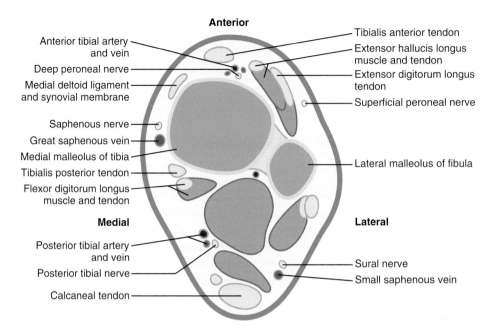

Fig. 5.5 The posterior tibial nerve courses medially between the Achilles tendon and the medial malleolus, where it divides into the medial and lateral plantar nerves, providing sensory innervation to the heel and medial plantar surface. (From Waldman S. *Atlas of Interventional Pain Management*. ed. 5. Philadelphia: Elsevier; 2021 [Fig. 147-3].)

accessible for neural blockade. The tibial nerve continues its downward course, running between the two heads of the gastrocnemius muscle, passing deep to the soleus muscle. The nerve courses medially between the Achilles tendon and the medial malleolus, where it divides into the medial and lateral plantar nerves, providing sensory innervation to the heel and medial plantar surface (Figs. 5.5 and 5.6). The tibial nerve is subject to compression at this point as the nerve passes through the posterior tarsal tunnel (Fig. 5.7). The posterior tarsal tunnel is made up of the flexor retinaculum, the bones of the ankle, and the lacunate ligament. In addition to the posterior tibial nerve, the tunnel contains the posterior tibial artery and vein as well as a number of flexor musculotendinous units (Fig. 5.8).

CLINICAL SYNDROME

Posterior tarsal tunnel syndrome is caused by compression of the posterior tibial nerve as it passes through the posterior tarsal tunnel. The posterior tarsal tunnel is made up of the flexor retinaculum, the bones of the ankle, and the lacunate ligament. In addition to the posterior tibial nerve, the tunnel contains the posterior tibial artery and certain flexor tendons that are subject to tenosynovitis. The most common cause of compression of the posterior tibial nerve at this location is

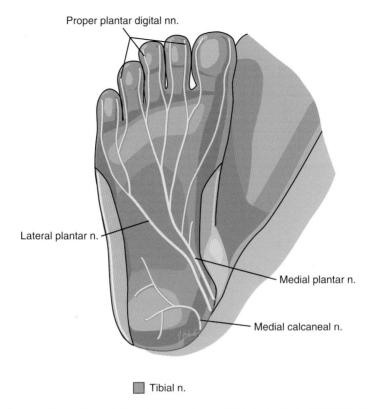

Fig. 5.6 Sensory innervation of the plantar surface of the foot. (From Waldman S. *Atlas of Interventional Pain Management*. ed. 5. Philadelphia: Elsevier; 2021 [Fig. 147-5].)

trauma to the ankle, including fracture, dislocation, and crush injury (Fig. 5.9). Thrombophlebitis involving the posterior tibial artery has also been implicated in the development of posterior tarsal tunnel syndrome, as has the wearing of tight high-heeled shoes with straps. Tumors of the posterior tibial nerve can also cause symptoms in the distribution of the posterior tibial nerve (Fig. 5.10). Patients with rheumatoid arthritis have a higher incidence of posterior tarsal tunnel syndrome than the general population. Posterior tarsal tunnel syndrome is much more common than anterior tarsal tunnel syndrome.

SIGNS AND SYMPTOMS

Posterior tarsal tunnel syndrome manifests in a manner analogous to carpal tunnel syndrome. Patients complain of pain, numbness, and paresthesias in the sole of the foot; these symptoms may also radiate proximal to the entrapment, into the medial ankle (see Fig. 5.7). Patients may note weakness of the toe flexors and

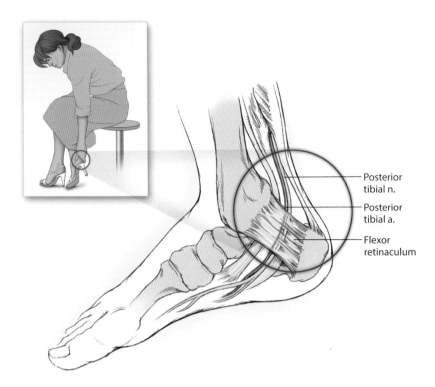

Fig. 5.7 The tibial nerve is subject to compression at this point as the nerve passes through the posterior tarsal tunnel. The posterior tarsal tunnel is made up of the flexor retinaculum, the bones of the ankle, and the lacunate ligament. (From Waldman S. *Atlas of Common Pain Syndromes*. ed. 4. Philadelphia: Elsevier; 2019 [Fig. 125-2].)

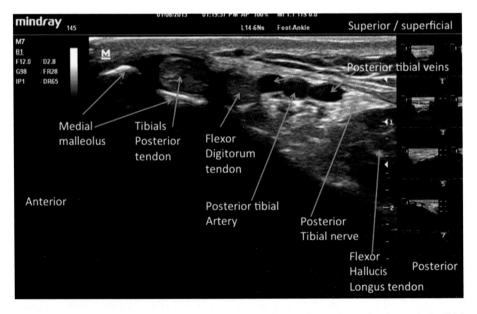

Fig. 5.8 In addition to the posterior tibial nerve, the posterior tarsal tunnel contains the posterior tibial artery and vein as well as a number of flexor musculotendinous units.

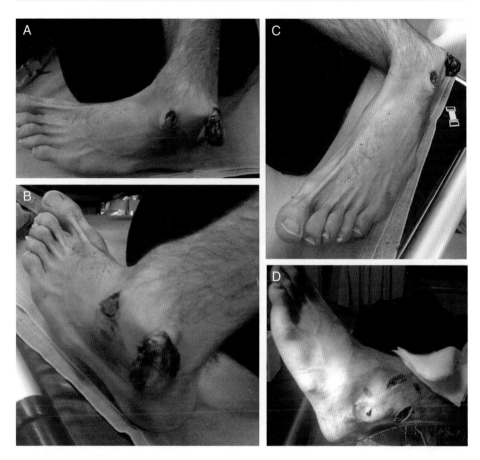

Fig. 5.9 Open posteromedial dislocation of the ankle status (A–C) before and (D) after reduction. (From Lazarettos I, Brilakis E, Efstathopoulos N. Open ankle dislocation without associated malleolar fracture. *J Foot Ankle Surg.* 2013;52(4):508–512 [Fig. 1]. ISSN 1067-2516, https://doi.org/10.1053/j.jfas.2013.03.017, http://www.sciencedirect.com/science/article/pii/S106725161300118X.)

instability of the foot resulting from weakness of the lumbrical muscles. Nighttime foot pain analogous to that of carpal tunnel syndrome is often present.

Physical findings include tenderness over the posterior tibial nerve at the medial malleolus. A positive Tinel sign just below and behind the medial malleolus over the posterior tibial nerve is usually present (see Fig. 5.2). Active inversion of the ankle often reproduces the symptoms of posterior tarsal tunnel syndrome. Medial and lateral plantar divisions of the posterior tibial nerve provide motor innervation to the intrinsic muscles of the foot. Thus, weakness of the flexor digitorum brevis and the lumbrical muscles may be present if these branches of the nerve are affected.

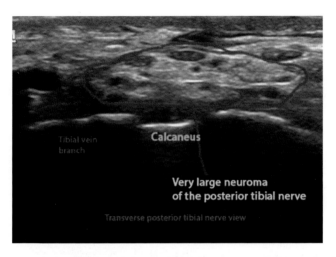

Fig. 5.10   Transverse ultrasound image demonstrating a large neuroma of the posterior tibial nerve.

TESTING

EMG can distinguish lumbar radiculopathy and diabetic polyneuropathy from posterior tarsal tunnel syndrome. Plain radiographs, magnetic resonance imaging (MRI), and ultrasound imaging are indicated for all patients who present with posterior tarsal tunnel syndrome to rule out occult bony disease (Figs. 5.11 and 5.12). MRI and ultrasound imaging of the ankle and foot are also indicated if joint instability or a space-occupying lesion is suspected (Fig. 5.13). Based on the patient's clinical presentation, additional testing may be warranted, including a complete blood count, uric acid level, erythrocyte sedimentation rate, and antinuclear antibody testing. The injection technique described later serves as both a diagnostic and a therapeutic maneuver.

DIFFERENTIAL DIAGNOSIS

Posterior tarsal tunnel syndrome is often misdiagnosed as arthritis of the ankle joint, lumbar radiculopathy, or diabetic polyneuropathy (Box 5.1). Patients with arthritis of the ankle, however, have radiographic evidence of arthritis. Most patients suffering from lumbar radiculopathy have reflex, motor, and sensory changes associated with back pain, whereas those with posterior tarsal tunnel syndrome have no reflex changes, and motor and sensory changes are limited to the distribution of the distal posterior tibial nerve. However, lumbar radiculopathy and posterior tibial nerve entrapment may coexist as the double crush syndrome. Diabetic polyneuropathy generally manifests as a symmetric sensory deficit involving the entire foot, rather than a condition limited to the

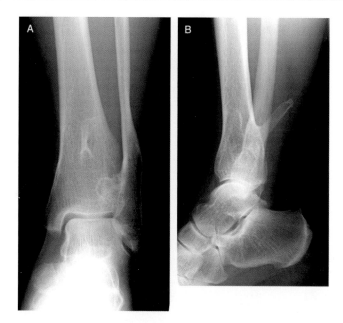

Fig. 5.11   Anteroposterior (A) and lateral (B) radiographs of the left ankle of a 52-year-old woman presenting with symptoms consistent with posterior tarsal tunnel syndrome. Note the presence of osteochondromas on both the distal tibia and fibula. (From Matsumoto K, Sumi H, Shimizu K. Tibial osteochondroma causing foot pain mimicking tarsal tunnel syndrome: a case report. *J Foot Ankle Surg.* 2005;44(2):159–162.)

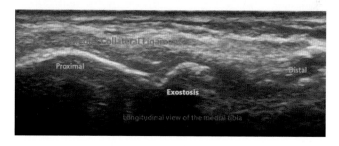

Fig. 5.12   Longitudinal ultrasound image on the medial tibia demonstrating an exostosis compressing the posterior tibial nerve.

distribution of the posterior tibial nerve. When posterior tarsal tunnel syndrome occurs in diabetic patients, diabetic polyneuropathy is usually also present.

TREATMENT

Mild cases of tarsal tunnel syndrome usually respond to conservative therapy; surgery should be reserved for severe cases. Initial treatment of tarsal tunnel

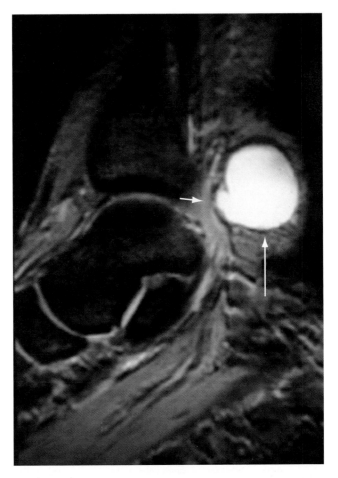

Fig. 5.13 Tarsal tunnel syndrome. Sagittal short tau inversion recovery magnetic resonance image shows a ganglion cyst *(long arrow)* compressing the neurovascular bundle in the tarsal tunnel *(short arrow)*. (From Edelman RR, Hesselink JR, Zlatkin MB, et al., eds. *Clinical Magnetic Resonance Imaging.* ed. 3. Philadelphia: Saunders; 2006:3454.)

syndrome consists of simple analgesics, nonsteroidal antiinflammatory drugs, or cyclooxygenase-2 inhibitors and splinting of the ankle. At a minimum, the splint should be worn at night, but wearing it for 24 hours a day is ideal. Avoidance of repetitive activities that may be responsible for the development of tarsal tunnel syndrome can also ameliorate the symptoms. If patients fail to respond to these conservative measures, injection of the tarsal tunnel with local anesthetic and steroid is a reasonable next step. Ultrasound needle guidance will improve the accuracy of needle placement and decrease the incidence of needle-related complications (Fig. 5.14).

BOX 5.1 ■ Conditions Associated With Posterior Tarsal Tunnel Syndrome

Structural/Anatomic
- Lipoma
- Ganglion
- Neuroma
- Aneurysm
- Dislocation
- Fracture

Inflammatory
- Tenosynovitis
- Collagen vascular disease
  - Rheumatoid arthritis
  - Scleroderma
- Gout

Neuropathic/Ischemic
- Diabetes
- Alcoholism
- Vitamin abnormalities
- Ischemic neuropathies
- Peripheral neuropathies
- Amyloidosis

Repetitive Stress Related
- Abnormal foot and ankle position
- Microtrauma
- Vibration

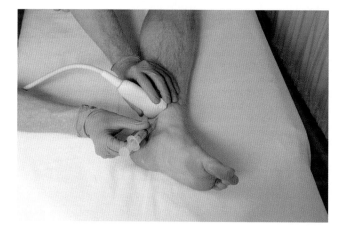

Fig. 5.14 Proper out-of-plane needle position for performing posterior tibial nerve block at the ankle.

HIGH-YIELD TAKEAWAYS

- The patient is afebrile, making an acute infectious etiology unlikely.
- The patient's symptomatology is thought to be the result of trauma to the right posterior tibial nerve at the ankle.
- Physical examination and testing should focus on identification of the various causes of posterior tarsal tunnel syndrome.
- The patient exhibits the neurologic and physical examination findings that are highly suggestive of posterior tarsal tunnel syndrome.
- The patient's symptoms are unilateral, suggestive of a local process rather than a systemic inflammatory process.
- Plain radiographs will provide high-yield information regarding the bony contents of the joint, but ultrasound imaging and MRI will be more useful in identifying soft tissue pathology that may be responsible for posterior tibial nerve compromise.
- EMG and nerve conduction velocity testing will help delineate the location and degree of nerve compromise if posterior tibial nerve compromise is suspected.

Suggested Readings

Fraser TW, Doty JF. Peripheral nerve blocks in foot and ankle surgery. *Orthop Clin North Am.* 2017;48(4):507–515.

Grant CRK, Raju PKBC. Lower limb nerve blocks. *Anaesth Intens Care Med.* 2016;17(4): 182–186.

Waldman SD. Posterior tarsal tunnel syndrome and other abnormalities of the posterior tibial nerve. In: *Waldman's Comprehensive Atlas of Diagnostic Ultrasound of Painful Conditions.* ed. 2. Philadelphia: Wolters Kluwer; 2016:952–963.

Waldman SD. Posterior tarsal tunnel syndrome. In: *Atlas of Common Pain Syndromes.* ed. 4. Philadelphia: Elsevier; 2019:496–499.

Waldman SD. The tibial nerve. In: *Pain Review.* ed. 2. Philadelphia: Saunders; 2017:131–133.

Waldman SD. Tibial nerve block at the knee. In: *Pain Review.* ed. 2. Philadelphia: Saunders; 2017:534–535.

Waldman SD, Campbell RSD. Posterior tarsal tunnel syndrome. In: *Imaging of Pain.* Philadelphia: Saunders Elsevier; 2010;425–426.

Paul Reckinger

A 32-Year-Old Real Estate Agent With Severe Right Ankle Pain With an Associated Catching Sensation

- Learn the common causes of ankle pain.
- Develop an understanding of the unique anatomy of the ankle joint.
- Develop an understanding of the musculotendinous units that surround the ankle joint.
- Develop an understanding of the anatomy of the Achilles tendon.
- Develop an understanding of the causes of Achilles tendinitis.
- Develop an understanding of the differential diagnosis of Achilles tendinitis.
- Learn the clinical presentation of Achilles tendinitis.
- Learn how to examine the ankle and Achilles tendon.
- Learn how to use physical examination to identify Achilles tendinitis.
- Develop an understanding of the treatment options for Achilles tendinitis.

Paul Reckinger

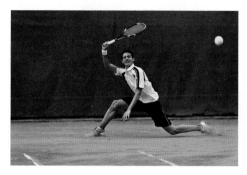

Paul Reckinger is a 32-year-old commercial real estate agent with the chief complaint of, "I have a catch in the back of my right ankle that hurts like hell." Paul stated that he recently competed in a tennis tournament at his country club and thought that was the reason for his ankle problem. "Doc, the competition was really brutal, but I gave it my all. I was up against this guy in the semifinals, and we were very evenly matched. The game went on for what seemed like hours, and neither of us could bring the game home. It was match point, and when I lunged for the ball I felt something in the back of my right ankle tear as I hit the ball. There was no way that guy was going to get to that ball the way I returned it, but from then on the back of my ankle has been hurting, especially in the mornings, when I first get up to go to the bathroom. Then I feel a catch and a sharp pain, and I have to hobble into the bathroom. It gets a little better after I'm up and on it for a while."

I asked Paul about any antecedent ankle trauma, and he said no. I asked what made the pain better, and he said a couple of Aleves washed down with a couple of single-malt whiskeys seemed to help. I asked Paul what made it worse, and he said the heating pad and walking up and down stairs. I asked how he was sleeping, and he said, "Not worth a crap. Every time I roll over, if I move my ankle, the pain wakes me up. I can't lie on my right side, and that's the side I like to sleep on." He denied fever and chills. I asked Paul to point with one finger to show me where it hurt the most. He pointed to the area above the posterior aspect of the right calcaneus.

On physical examination, Paul was afebrile. His respirations were 16, and his pulse was 72 and regular. He was normotensive with a blood pressure of 120/70. Paul's head, eyes, ears, nose, throat (HEENT) exam was normal. His cardiopulmonary examination was completely normal. His thyroid was normal, as was his abdominal examination, which revealed no abnormal mass or organomegaly. There was no costovertebral angle (CVA) tenderness, nor was there any peripheral edema. Paul's low back examination was unremarkable. Visual inspection of the right ankle was normal. I asked Paul to get up and walk, and he walked with a flat-footed gait to avoid plantarflexing his foot. The area over the distal Achilles tendon was a little warm, but it did not appear to be infected. There was marked tenderness to palpation of the distal Achilles tendon, and I perceived a creaking sensation when I asked Paul to plantarflex his foot (Fig. 6.1). Paul's pain was reproduced with resisted plantarflexion of the foot. There was pain to externally rotate his ankle. The left ankle examination was

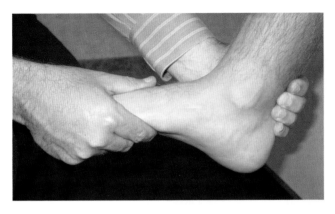

Fig. 6.1   Eliciting the creak sign for Achilles tendinitis. (From Waldman SD. *Physical Diagnosis of Pain: An Atlas of Signs and Symptoms*. Philadelphia: Saunders; 2006:377.)

normal, as was examination of his other major joints. A careful neurologic exami-nation of the upper extremities revealed no evidence of peripheral or entrapment neuropathy, and the deep tendon reflexes were normal.

Key Clinical Points—What's Important and What's Not

THE HISTORY

- History of acute trauma to the posterior ankle following lunging for a ball while playing tennis
- No history of previous significant ankle pain
- No fever or chills
- Acute onset of ankle pain following a traumatic event with exacerbation of pain with ankle use
- Pain in the right ankle
- A catching sensation when walking
- Sleep disturbance

THE PHYSICAL EXAMINATION

- Patient is afebrile
- Tenderness to palpation of the distal Achilles tendon
- Palpation of the right Achilles tendon reveals warmth to touch
- Creaking sensation when palpating the right Achilles tendon during passive plantarflexion of the foot
- Increased pain with resisted plantarflexion of the right foot and ankle

- No evidence of infection
- Flat-footed gait in an effort to splint the inflamed Achilles tendon

OTHER FINDINGS OF NOTE

- Normal HEENT examination
- Normal cardiovascular examination
- Normal pulmonary examination
- Normal abdominal examination
- No peripheral edema
- Normal upper extremity neurologic examination, motor and sensory examination
- Examination of joints other than the right ankle was normal

 What Tests Would You Like to Order?

The following tests were ordered:
- Plain radiographs of the right ankle
- Ultrasound of the right ankle, including the Achilles tendon

TEST RESULTS

The plain radiographs of the right ankle revealed a significantly calcified insertion of the Achilles tendon with Haglund deformity (Fig. 6.2).

Ultrasound examination of the right Achilles tendon reveals bruising of the Achilles tendon from direct trauma as well as extensive tendinosis with significant tearing of the tendon substance (Fig. 6.3).

 Clinical Correlation—Putting It All Together

What is the diagnosis?
- Achilles tendinitis

The Science Behind the Diagnosis
ANATOMY

The Achilles tendon is the thickest and strongest tendon in the body, yet is also very susceptible to rupture. The common tendon of the gastrocnemius muscle, the Achilles tendon begins at midcalf and continues downward to attach to the

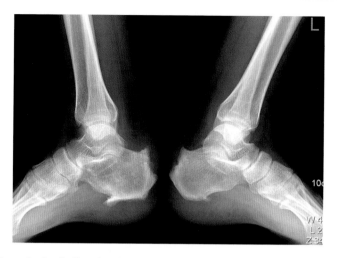

Fig. 6.2 Radiograph of a significantly calcified insertional Achilles tendon with Haglund deformity. (From Miao X-D, Jiang H, Wu Y-P, et al. Treatment of calcified insertional Achilles tendinopathy by the posterior midline approach. *J Foot Ankle Surg.* 2016;55(3):529–534 [Fig. 1]. ISSN 1067-2516, https://doi.org/10.1053/j.jfas.2016.01.016, http://www.sciencedirect.com/science/article/pii/S106725161600017X.)

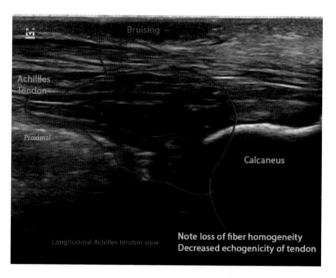

Fig. 6.3 Longitudinal ultrasound image demonstrating bruising of the Achilles tendon from direct trauma as well as extensive tendinosis with significant tearing of the tendon substance.

posterior calcaneus, where it may become inflamed (Fig. 6.4). The Achilles tendon narrows during this downward course, becoming most narrow at approximately 5 cm above its calcaneal insertion. It is at this narrowest point that tendinitis also may occur. A bursa is located between the Achilles tendon and

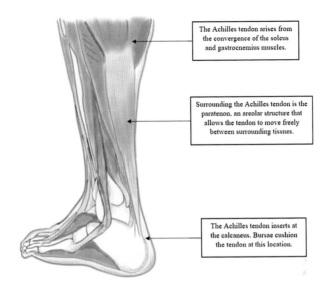

The Achilles tendon arises from the convergence of the soleus and gastrocnemius muscles.

Surrounding the Achilles tendon is the paratenon, an areolar structure that allows the tendon to move freely between surrounding tissues.

The Achilles tendon inserts at the calcaneus. Bursae cushion the tendon at this location.

Fig. 6.4 The Achilles tendon is the thickest and strongest tendon in the body, yet is also very susceptible to rupture. The common tendon of the gastrocnemius muscle, the Achilles tendon begins at midcalf and continues downward to attach to the posterior calcaneus. (From Fares M, Khachfe H, Salhab H, et al. Achilles tendinopathy: exploring injury characteristics and current treatment modalities. *Foot.* 2021;46 [Fig. 1].)

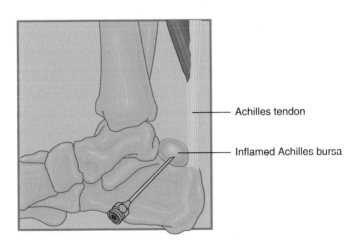

Achilles tendon

Inflamed Achilles bursa

Fig. 6.5 The Achilles bursa. (From Waldman S. *Atlas of Pain Management Injection Techniques.* ed. 4. St. Louis: Elsevier; 2017 [Fig. 168-1].)

the base of the tibia and the upper posterior calcaneus (Fig. 6.5). This bursa also may become inflamed as a result of coexistent Achilles tendinitis and may confuse the clinical picture.

CLINICAL SYNDROME

Achilles tendinitis has become more common as jogging has increased in popularity. The Achilles tendon is susceptible to the development of tendinitis both at its insertion on the calcaneus and at its narrowest part, a point approximately 5 cm above its insertion. The Achilles tendon is subjected to repetitive motion that may result in microtrauma, which heals poorly owing to the tendon's avascular nature. The appearance of Achilles tendinitis has been described as having a "crabmeat" appearance owing to the nonlinear orientation of the tendon fibers (Fig. 6.6). Running is often the inciting factor in acute Achilles tendinitis, which frequently coexists with bursitis and thus causes additional pain and functional disability. Calcium deposition around the tendon may occur if inflammation

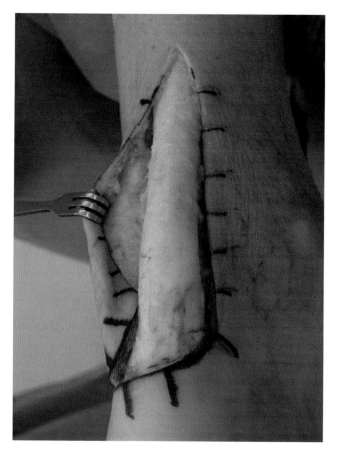

Fig. 6.6 Bulbous "crabmeat" tendon without distinct orientation in the central aspect of the Achilles tendon. (From Sundararajan PP. Transosseous fixation in insertional Achilles tendonitis. *J Foot Ankle Surg.* 2012;51(6):806–812.)

persists, and this complication makes subsequent treatment more difficult. Continued trauma to the inflamed tendon may ultimately result in tendon rupture.

SIGNS AND SYMPTOMS

The onset of Achilles tendinitis is usually acute, occurring after overuse or misuse of the ankle joint. Inciting activities include running with sudden stops and starts, such as when playing tennis. Improper stretching of the gastrocnemius and Achilles tendon before exercise has also been implicated in Achilles tendinitis, as well as in acute tendon rupture. The pain of Achilles tendinitis is constant and severe and is localized in the posterior ankle (Fig. 6.7). Significant sleep disturbance is often reported. Patients may attempt to splint the inflamed Achilles tendon by adopting a flat-footed gait to avoid plantarflexing the tendon. Pain is induced with resisted plantarflexion of the foot, and a creaking or grating sensation may be palpated when the foot is passively plantarflexed (see Fig. 6.2). A

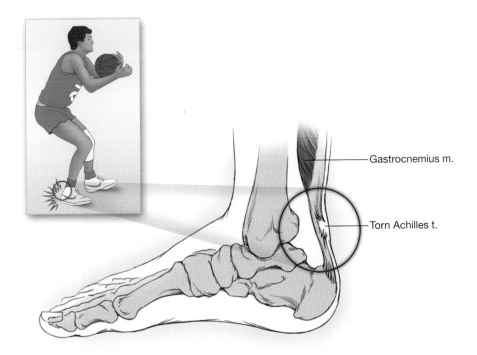

Gastrocnemius m.

Torn Achilles t.

Fig. 6.7 The pain of Achilles tendinitis is constant and severe and is localized to the posterior ankle. (From Waldman S. *Atlas of Common Pain Syndromes*. ed. 4. Philadelphia: Elsevier; 2019 [Fig. 126-2].)

chronically inflamed Achilles tendon may suddenly rupture from stress or during injection into the tendon itself.

TESTING

Plain radiographs, ultrasound imaging, and magnetic resonance imaging (MRI) are indicated in all patients who present with posterior ankle pain (Figs. 6.8 and 6.9). Color Doppler may help identify neovascularity of the tendon that is highly suggestive of tendinitis (Fig. 6.10). MRI and ultrasound imaging of the ankle are also indicated if joint instability is suspected. Radionuclide bone scanning and computerized tomography (CT) is useful to identify stress fractures not seen on plain radiographs (Fig. 6.11). Based on the patient's clinical presentation, additional testing may be warranted, including a complete blood count, erythrocyte sedimentation rate, comprehensive metabolic profile, and antinuclear antibody testing. Injection of the inflamed Achilles tendon with local anesthetic and steroid serves as both a diagnostic and a therapeutic maneuver (Fig. 6.12).

DIFFERENTIAL DIAGNOSIS

Achilles tendinitis is usually easily identified on clinical grounds. However, if the bursa located between the Achilles tendon and the base of

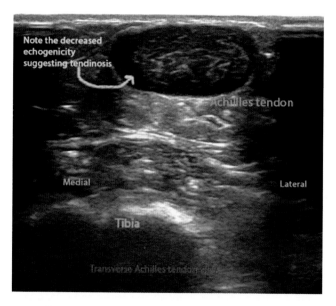

Fig. 6.8 Transverse ultrasound image demonstrating tendinosis of the Achilles tendon. Note decreased echogenicity.

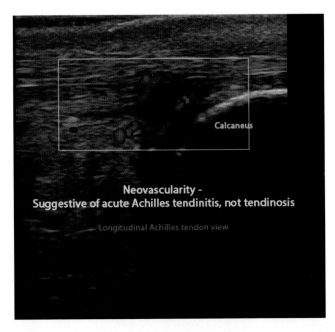

Fig. 6.9   Color Doppler may help identify neovascularity of the tendon that is highly suggestive of tendinitis.

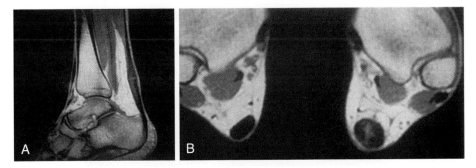

Fig. 6.10   Magnetic resonance imaging of chronic degenerative tendinosis with thickening of the Achilles tendon in the sagittal (A) and coronal (B) planes compared with the opposite Achilles tendon. (From Lesic A, Bumbasirevic M. Disorders of the Achilles tendon. *Curr Orthop*. 2004;18(1):63—75.)

the tibia and the upper posterior calcaneus is inflamed, coexistent bursitis may confuse the diagnosis. Stress fractures of the ankle may also mimic Achilles tendinitis.

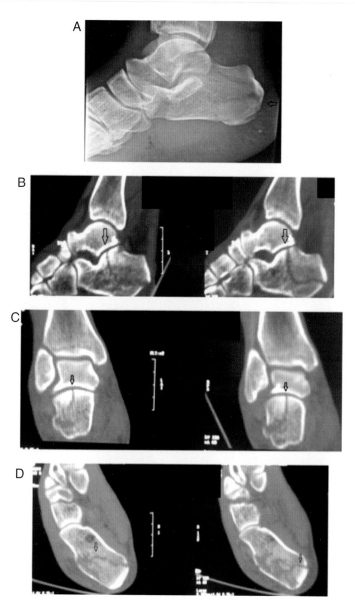

Fig. 6.11 A 33-year-old male patient presenting after a fall from a height. Plain x-ray and computed tomography (CT) showed an intraarticular fracture (Sanders type I) of the right calcaneus. (A) Lateral radiograph showed a fracture line of the right calcaneal body extending into the subtalar joint *(arrow)*. (B) Sagittal multidetector CT scan of the right foot revealed a fracture of the right calcaneal body extending into the subtalar joint *(arrows)*. (C) Coronal multidetector CT scan of the right foot showed an undisplaced fracture that involved the posterior facet of the subtalar joint *(arrows)*. (D) Axial multidetector CT scan showed a calcaneal fracture with no calcaneocuboid joint involvement *(arrows)*. (From Moussa KM, Hassaan MAE, Moharram AN, et al. The role of multidetector CT in evaluation of calcaneal fractures. *Egypt J Radiol Nucl Med.* 2015;46(2):413–421 [Fig. 2]. ISSN 0378-603X, https://doi.org/10.1016/j.ejrnm.2015.02.013, http://www.sciencedirect.com/science/article/pii/S0378603X15000571.)

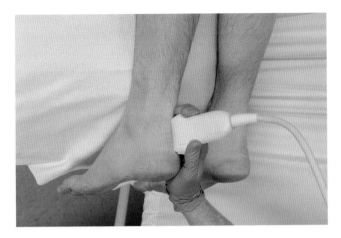

Fig. 6.12   Proper position of the ultrasound transducer for the injection of Achilles tendinitis.

TREATMENT

Initial treatment of the pain and functional disability associated with Achilles tendinitis includes a combination of nonsteroidal antiinflammatory drugs (NSAIDs) or cyclooxygenase-2 inhibitors and physical therapy. The local application of heat and cold may also be beneficial. Repetitive activities thought to be responsible for the development of tendinitis, such as jogging, should be avoided. For patients who do not respond to these treatment modalities, injection with local anesthetic and steroid is a reasonable next step.

Physical modalities, including local heat and gentle range-of-motion exercises, should be introduced several days after the patient undergoes injection. Vigorous exercises should be avoided because they will exacerbate the patient's symptoms. Simple analgesics and NSAIDs can be used concurrently with this injection technique. Ultrasound needle guidance will improve the accuracy of needle placement and decrease the incidence of needle-related complications. The injection of platelet-rich plasma and/or stem cells may reduce the pain and functional disability of Achilles tendinitis

HIGH-YIELD TAKEAWAYS

- The patient is afebrile, making an acute infectious etiology (e.g., septic arthritis) unlikely.
- The patient's symptomatology is the result of acute trauma, and physical examination and testing should focus on identification of occult fractures,

(Continued)

bursitis, or other pathology that might mimic the clinical presentation of Achilles tendinitis.

- The patient has tenderness over the distal Achilles, which is highly suggestive of Achilles tendinitis.
- There is warmth over the distal Achilles tendon, which supports the diagnosis of tendinitis.
- The patient's symptoms are unilateral and involve only one joint, which is more suggestive of a local process than a systemic polyarthropathy.
- Sleep disturbance is common and must be addressed concurrently with the patient's pain symptomatology.
- Plain radiographs and CT scanning will provide high-yield information regarding the bony contents of the joint, but ultrasound imaging and MRI will be more useful in identifying soft tissue pathology.

Suggested Readings

Kim YC, Ahn JH, Kim MS. Infectious Achilles tendinitis after local injection of human placental extracts: a case report. *J Foot Ankle Surg.* 2015;54(6):1193–1196.

Tenforde AS, Yin A, Hunt KJ. Foot and ankle injuries in runners. *Phys Med Rehabil Clin N Am.* 2016;27(1):121–137.

Waldman SD. Achilles tendinitis and other abnormalities of the Achilles tendon. In: *Waldman's Comprehensive Atlas of Diagnostic Ultrasound of Painful Conditions.* ed. 2. Phildelphia: Wolters Kluwer; 2016:986–996.

Waldman SD. Achilles tendon injection. In: *Atlas of Pain Management Injection Techniques.* ed. 4. Philadelphia: Elsevier; 2017:633–636.

Waldman SD. The Achilles tendon. In: *Pain Review.* ed. 2. Philadelphia: Elsevier; 2017:153–154.

Waldman SD, Campbell RSD. Achilles tendinitis. In: *Imaging of Pain.* ed. 1. Philadelphia: Saunders; 2011:427–430.

Waldman SD, Campbell RSD. Anatomy: special imaging considerations of the ankle and foot. In: *Imaging of Pain.* ed. 1. Philadelphia: Saunders; 2011:417–420.

Weinfeld SB. Achilles tendon disorders. *Med Clin North Am.* 2014;98(2):331–338.

DeShawn Freely

A 29-Year-Old Basketball Player With the Feeling He Had Been Shot in the Ankle

- Learn the common causes of ankle pain.
- Develop an understanding of the unique anatomy of the ankle joint.
- Develop an understanding of the anatomy of the Achilles tendon and gastrocnemius muscle.
- Understand the function of the Achilles tendon.
- Develop an understanding of the causes of Achilles tendon rupture.
- Develop an understanding of the various types of Achilles tendon pathology.
- Learn the clinical presentation of Achilles tendon rupture.
- Learn how to examine the Achilles tendon.
- Learn how to use physical examination to identify pathology of the Achilles tendon.
- Develop an understanding of the treatment options for Achilles tendon rupture.

DeShawn Freeley

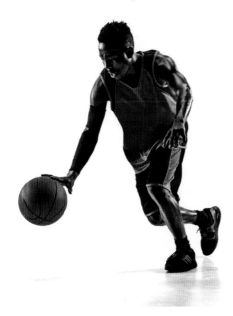

DeShawn Freeley is a 29-year-old basketball player with the chief complaint of, "I feel like somebody shot me in the back of my ankle, and now I can barely walk." I asked, "DeShawn, tell me exactly what happened." He responded, "My wife keeps telling me it's time to retire, but what am I going to do, sell insurance? I was going for a lay-up, and some kid with more muscle than brains came smashing into me when I was coming down. I made the basket, but he knocked me sideways, and I was really off balance when I landed. I landed really hard, and it sounded like somebody shot a gun. A second later I feel this unbelievable pain in the back of my ankle. Honestly, Doctor, for a second or two, I thought that I had actually been shot, but as soon as I got to my feet, I knew exactly what happened. I've seen it in other players before. I had a big bruise on the back of my ankle and the side of my foot. They helped me to the locker room, and I just sat there while the trainer put some ice on it—like that was going to help. Doctor, I felt like crying. I just sat there. And on top of it, we lost the game and our chance for the playoffs. I knew there was going to be a lot of 'I told you so' comments when Amy—that's my wife—found out." I broke in and asked, "DeShawn, had your ankle been bothering you before you injured it?" He shook his head and looked at me like I was stupid, and said, "Doc, have you ever played basketball for a living?" He then smiled and looked me up and down, and said, "I guess not. I may look like 10 miles of bad road, but I had another season or two in me. I've stayed in shape, stayed off the drugs, and tried to eat right."

I asked DeShawn how he was sleeping, and he said that as long as he didn't lie on his bad leg, it was lights out and sweet dreams. DeShawn denied any fever or chills associated with his pain. I asked if he had taken any antibiotics recently, and with an surprised look, DeShawn said, "Doc, are you a mind reader or something? About a month ago, we were on the road and I picked up a cough, and the team doctor put me on some Cipro. It put me right after a couple of days. I played through it. Like I said, I'm tough." I asked, "Tell me about your walking." He replied, "Doc, I can get around, but it's almost impossible to walk stairs."

On physical examination, DeShawn was afebrile. His respirations were 18, and his pulse was 64 and regular. His blood pressure was 148/90. His head, eyes, ears, nose, throat (HEENT) exam was normal, as was his cardiopulmonary examination. His thyroid was normal. His abdominal examination revealed no abnormal mass or organomegaly. There was a small right lower quadrant scar that DeShawn said was from having his appendix removed when he was in high school. There was no costovertebral angle (CVA) tenderness or peripheral edema. His low back examination was unremarkable. Visual inspection of the right ankle revealed a large area of ecchymosis over the lower calf and over the arch of his foot. I asked DeShawn to point with one finger to show me where it hurt the most. He pointed to the area just above the superior margin of the calcaneous. Before I could go on, he pointed to the bulge in his right calf and said, "Doc, let's not worry about the pain. You need to get this tendon put back together." I said to DeShawn, "I know exactly what it is and I know exactly what to do about it. So I got this! Let me make sure nothing else is going on, then together we will map out a plan." He smiled weakly and said, "You're the doctor."

I then asked DeShawn to stand up and place both feet flat on the floor. I asked him to stand on his tiptoes. As expected, his toe raise test for Achilles tendon rupture was positive on the right (Fig. 7.1A). I then asked DeShawn to get back on the examination table and hang his legs over the edge. As expected, the Thompson squeeze test was positive (see Fig. 7.1B). I had DeShawn roll over on his stomach and flex his knees to 90 degrees; not surprisingly, he was unable to plantarflex the affected lower extremity (Fig. 7.2). He was tender over the distal Achilles tendon and a tendon defect was easily identifiable, as was the proximal bunching of the gastrocnemius muscle. Passive range of motion of the right ankle was normal. DeShawn's left ankle examination was normal, as was examination of his other major joints. A careful neurologic examination of the upper and lower extremities revealed no evidence of peripheral or entrapment neuropathy, and the deep tendon reflexes were normal.

I told DeShawn that I was pretty sure that kid had got the better of him, and suspected he had ruptured his Achilles tendon. He was going to need surgery to repair it. I told him that I want to get some confirmatory testing to ascertain the condition of the proximal tendon so we could better go in and sew it all back together.

DeShawn slowly shook his head, and as a tear coursed down his cheek, he said, "You know, Doc, I had a pretty good run. I knew it wouldn't be forever, but I thought I had a couple more seasons. Let's get this fixed." He was so down I decided to wait until after surgery to tell him about the role that the Cipro may have played in his tendon rupture.

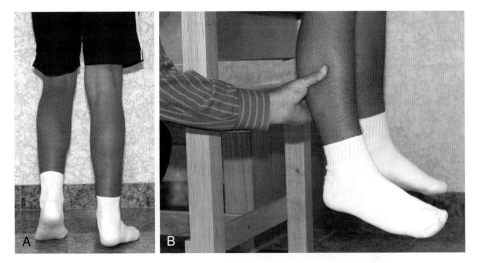

Fig. 7.1   (A) To perform the toe raise test for Achilles tendon rupture, the patient is asked to stand in a comfortable position and then to raise oneself on tiptoe. (B) To perform the Thompson squeeze test for Achilles tendon rupture, the examiner grasps the calf on the patient's affected side just below the point of the calf's maximum girth and firmly squeezes the calf. Absence of plantarflexion on the affected side provides a presumptive diagnosis of rupture of the Achilles tendon. (From Waldman SD. *Physical Diagnosis of Pain: An Atlas of Signs and Symptoms*. 2. Philadelphia: Saunders; 2010:344, 346.)

Key Clinical Points—What's Important and What's Not

THE HISTORY

- History of sudden onset of pain in the posterior ankle with an associated cosmetic deformity
- History of sudden, audible pop in the ankle at the time of the acute injury
- History of significant ecchymosis over the posterior ankle and arch of the foot
- No history of previous significant ankle injury
- No fever or chills
- Sleep disturbance

THE PHYSICAL EXAMINATION

- Patient is afebrile
- Palpation of right ankle reveals tenderness over the Achilles tendon
- Presence of significant ecchymosis over the posterior ankle and arch of the affected foot
- Palpable defect in the Achilles tendon
- Normal passive range of motion of the right ankle

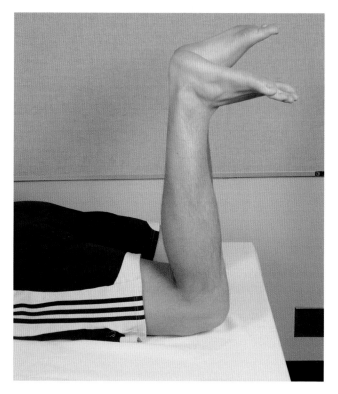

Fig. 7.2   To perform the Matles test for Achilles tendon rupture, the patient is placed in the prone position, and the examiner passively flexes the patient's knees to 90 degrees while both of the patient's
feet are in neutral position. If the Achilles tendon is ruptured, there will be no plantarflexion of the
affected foot. (From Waldman S. *Physical Diagnosis of Pain: An Atlas of Signs and Symptoms*. ed. 4.
Philadelphia: Elsevier; 2021 [Fig. 274-1].)

- Positive toe raise test for Achilles tendon rupture (see Fig. 7.1A)
- Positive Thompson squeeze test for Achilles tendon rupture (see Fig. 7.1B)
- Positive Matles test for Achilles tendon rupture (see Fig. 7.2)

OTHER FINDINGS OF NOTE

- Normal HEENT examination
- Normal cardiovascular examination
- Normal pulmonary examination
- Normal abdominal examination with a well-healed appendectomy scar
  noted
- No peripheral edema
- Normal upper extremity neurologic examination, motor and sensory
  examination
- Examination of other joints was normal

What Tests Would You Like to Order?

The following tests were ordered:
- Plain radiographs of the ankle and foot
- Magnetic resonance imaging (MRI) of the right ankle to ascertain the condition of the distal Achilles tendon
- Ultrasound of the right ankle with special attention to the distal Achilles tendon

TEST RESULTS

Plain radiographs of the ankle and foot revealed no evidence of fracture but loss of equinus (Fig. 7.3).

MRI revealed distal and proximal ruptures in the watershed region of the Achilles tendon with central calcification (Fig. 7.4).

Ultrasound of the right Achilles tendon revealed a complete rupture of the Achilles tendon (Fig. 7.5).

Clinical Correlation—Putting It All Together

What is the diagnosis?
- Rupture of the Achilles tendon

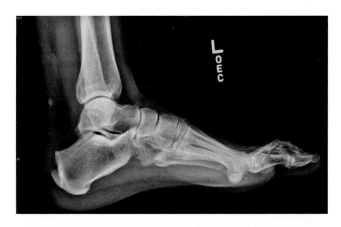

Fig. 7.3 Lateral radiograph showing calcification within the Achilles tendon and at the insertion. Note the lack of equinus in this nonweightbearing view. (From Saxena A, Hofer D. Triple Achilles tendon rupture: case report. *J Foot Ankle Surg*. 2018;57(2):404−408 [Fig. 1]. ISSN 1067-2516, https://doi.org/10.1053/j. jfas.2017.08.023, http://www.sciencedirect.com/science/article/pii/S1067251617305367.)

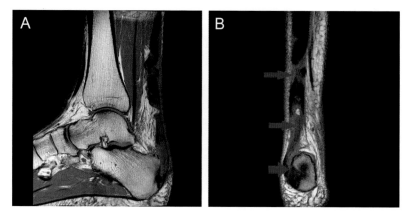

Fig. 7.4   (A) Lateral T1 magnetic resonance imaging (MRI) scan showing avulsion and distal and proximal ruptures in the dysvascular watershed region of the tendon with central calcification. (B) Coronal MRI scan showing same findings seen on lateral view and midsubstance calcification. (From Saxena A, Hofer D. Triple Achilles tendon rupture: case report. *J Foot Ankle Surg*. 2018;57(2):404−408 [Fig. 2]. ISSN 1067-2516, https://doi.org/10.1053/j.jfas.2017.08.023, http://www.sciencedirect.com/science/article/pii/S1067251617305367.)

The Science Behind the Diagnosis

ANATOMY OF THE ACHILLES TENDON

The Achilles tendon is the thickest and strongest tendon in the body, yet it is also very susceptible to rupture. The common tendon of the gastrocnemius muscle, the Achilles tendon begins at midcalf and continues downward to attach to the posterior calcaneus, where it may become inflamed (Fig. 7.6). The Achilles tendon narrows during this downward course, becoming most narrow at approximately 5 cm above its calcaneal insertion. It is at this narrowest point that tendinitis also may occur. A bursa is located between the Achilles tendon and the base of the tibia and the upper posterior calcaneus. This bursa also may become inflamed as a result of coexistent Achilles tendinitis and may confuse the clinical picture.

CLINICAL CONSIDERATIONS

Achilles tendon rupture most often occurs following an injury after acute push-off during jumping or sprinting as the result of extreme ankle dorsiflexion. Occurring in otherwise healthy adults, it is a disease of the third to fifth decades and has a male predominance. Rupture of the Achilles tendon most often occurs in the left leg because right-handed individuals usually push off with the left leg when they jump.

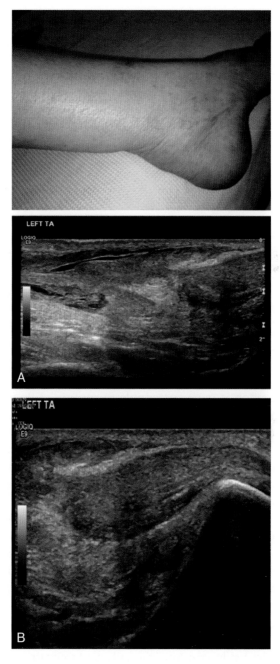

Fig. 7.5 Photograph of ankle in patient with complete rupture of the Achilles tendon. Note the obvious defect in the tendon. (A, B) Longitudinal ultrasound images demonstrating complete rupture of the Achilles tendon. (From AL-Saadi S, Michael A. Levofloxacin-induced Achilles tendinitis and tendon rupture. *Eur Geriatr Med*. 2012;3(6):380–381 [Fig. 1].)

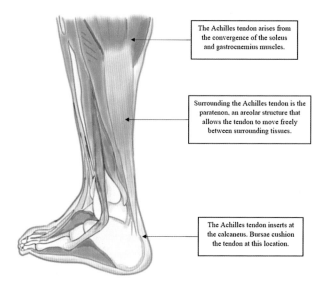

The Achilles tendon arises from the convergence of the soleus and gastrocnemius muscles.

Surrounding the Achilles tendon is the paratenon, an areolar structure that allows the tendon to move freely between surrounding tissues.

The Achilles tendon inserts at the calcaneus. Bursae cushion the tendon at this location.

Fig. 7.6 The Achilles tendon is the thickest and strongest tendon in the body, yet it is also very susceptible to rupture. The common tendon of the gastrocnemius muscle, the Achilles tendon begins at midcalf and continues downward to attach to the posterior calcaneus. (From Fares M, Khachfe H, Salhab H, et al. Achilles tendinopathy: exploring injury characteristics and current treatment modalities. *Foot*. 2021;46:101715 [Fig. 1].)

The Achilles tendon is most susceptible to rupture at its narrowest part, a point approximately 5 cm above its insertion (Fig. 7.7). The Achilles tendon is subjected to repetitive motion that may result in microtrauma, which heals poorly owing to the tendon's avascular nature. The repeated microtrauma leads to tendinitis and tendinopathy that may predispose the tendon to rupture. Achilles tendinitis frequently coexists with bursitis, which causes additional pain and functional disability.

In addition to traumatic rupture of the Achilles tendon, sudden nontraumatic rupture may occur. Factors that predispose the patient to traumatic and nontraumatic rupture of the Achilles tendon include steroid use, dialysis, gout, rheumatoid arthritis, systemic lupus erythematosus, diabetes, endocrinopathies, renal transplant, hyperlipidemias, and the use of fluoroquinolones (Box 7.1).

SIGNS AND SYMPTOMS

The onset of Achilles tendon rupture is usually acute, occurring after acute push-off during jumping or sprinting as the result of extreme ankle dorsiflexion. Improper stretching of the gastrocnemius and Achilles tendon before exercise has also been implicated in the development of Achilles tendinitis and acute tendon rupture. The pain of Achilles tendon rupture is constant and severe and is

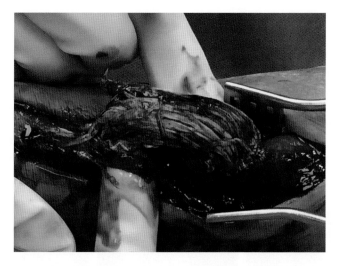

Fig. 7.7 Intraoperative view showing the watershed region ruptures. Calcification within the main body was palpable. (From Saxena A, Hofer D. Triple Achilles tendon rupture: case report. *J Foot Ankle Surg.* 2018;57(2):404–408 [Fig. 3]. ISSN 1067-2516, https://doi.org/10.1053/j.jfas.2017.08.023.)

BOX 7.1 ■ Factors Associated With Rupture of the Achilles Tendon

- Steroid use
- Dialysis
- Gout
- Rheumatoid arthritis
- Systemic lupus erythematosus
- Diabetes
- Thyroid disease
- Parathyroid disorders
- Endocrinopathies
- Renal transplantation
- Hyperlipidemias
- Fluoroquinolone use

---

localized in the posterior ankle. The patient often complains of a feeling like being kicked in the ankle. Significant ecchymosis, swelling, and hematoma are frequently present. Palpation of the ruptured Achilles tendon may reveal a lack of tendon continuity. The patient suffering from Achilles tendon rupture exhibits positive results of the toe raise and Thompson squeeze tests (see Fig. 7.1). The Matles knee flexion test can also help identify a ruptured Achilles tendon (see Fig. 7.2).

TESTING

Plain radiographs, ultrasound imaging, and MRI are indicated in all patients who present with posterior ankle pain and who are suspected of suffering from Achilles tendon rupture (Fig. 7.8). MRI of the ankle is also indicated if joint instability, bursitis, infection, or occult tumor is suspected (Fig. 7.9). Radionuclide bone scanning and computerized tomography are useful to identify stress fractures not seen on plain radiographs. Ultrasound imaging may also help assess the integrity of the Achilles tendon (see Fig. 7.8). Intraoperative plain radiographs can help

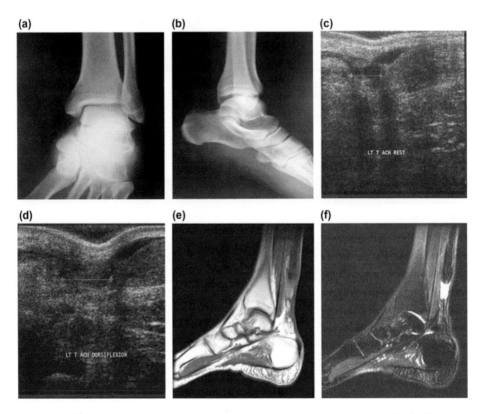

Fig. 7.8 (a, b) Plain x-ray anteroposterior and lateral views normal. (c) Longitudinal ultrasound images of the left Achilles tendon at rest showing complete rupture of the tendon. The gap between two stumps is seen filled with unclear fluid. (d) Longitudinal ultrasound images of the left Achilles tendon during dorsiflexion showing complete rupture of the tendon with widening of the gap between the two stumps. (e) Sagittal T1-weighted and (f) sagittal STIR-weighted image showing discontinuity of whole fibers of the distal third of tendo-Achilles with retraction and thickening of both torn ends leading to a gap *(arrow)* at the site of tear. This gap displays intermediate signal intensity in sagittal T1-weighted and hyperintense signal in sagittal STIR. (From Ibrahim NMAM, Elsaeed HH. Lesions of the Achilles tendon: evaluation with ultrasonography and magnetic resonance imaging. *Egypt J Radiol Nucl Med.* 2013;44(3):581–587 [Fig. 3]. ISSN 0378-603X, https://doi.org/10.1016/j.ejrnm.2013.05.006, http://www.sciencedirect.com/science/article/pii/S0378603X13000673.)

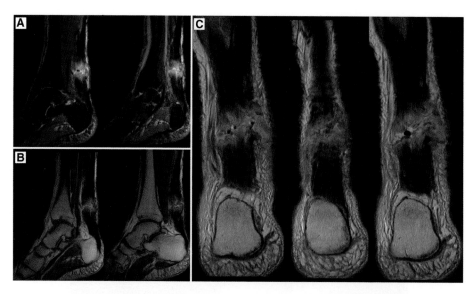

Fig. 7.9 Magnetic resonance scans of the right lower leg of the patient (postcontrast fat-suppressed T2-weighted sagittal views in A, T1-weighted sagittal views in B, and T1-weighted coronal views in C) demonstrating a complete tendon discontinuity 5.5 cm proximally to the insertion with a 1.3-cm gap and extensive postcontrast peripheral enhancement of soft tissues around the rupture site, consistent with deep infection. (From de Cesar Netto C, Bernasconi A, Roberts L, et al. Open re-rupture of the Achilles tendon following minimally invasive repair: a case report. *J Foot Ankle Surg.* 2018;57 (6):1272–1277 [Fig. 3]. ISSN 1067-2516, https://doi.org/10.1053/j.jfas.2018.04.002, http://www.sciencedirect.com/science/article/pii/S1067251618301546.)

demonstrate the reestablishment of appropriate heel tension by demonstrating return of equinus (Fig. 7.10; see Fig. 7.3 for comparison). Based on the patient's clinical presentation, additional testing may be warranted, including a complete blood count, comprehensive metabolic panel, erythrocyte sedimentation rate, and antinuclear antibody testing.

DIFFERENTIAL DIAGNOSIS

Achilles tendon rupture is usually easily identified on clinical grounds. However, if the bursa located between the Achilles tendon and the base of the tibia and the upper posterior calcaneus is inflamed, coexistent bursitis may confuse the diagnosis. Stress fractures of the ankle may also mimic the pain of Achilles tendon rupture (Fig. 7.11).

TREATMENT

Initial treatment of the pain and functional disability associated with Achilles tendon rupture includes elevation, relative rest, and ice. A combination of

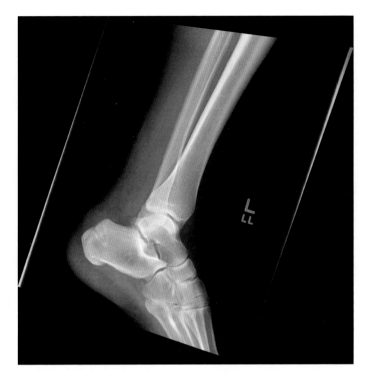

Fig. 7.10 Postoperative radiograph showing reestablishment of heel tension (equinus), drill holes for anchors, and removal of calcified Achilles tendon. (From Saxena A, Hofer D. Triple Achilles tendon rupture: case report. *J Foot Ankle Surg.* 2018;57(2):404−408 [Fig. 6]. ISSN 1067-2516, https://doi.org/10.1053/j.jfas.2017.08.023, http://www.sciencedirect.com/science/article/pii/S1067251617305367.)

nonsteroidal antiinflammatory drugs or cyclooxygenase-2 inhibitors and short-acting opioid analgesics, such as hydrocodone, may be necessary to manage the acute pain associated with this condition. Although some specialists recommend conservative therapy, most believe that surgical repair of the tendon with postoperative immobilization is the best option in otherwise healthy patients (see Fig. 7.6). Clinical experience suggests that the injection of platelet-rich plasma and/or stem cells may improve tendon healing.

HIGH-YIELD TAKEAWAYS

- The patient is afebrile, making an acute infectious etiology (e.g., septic arthritis) unlikely.

(Continued)

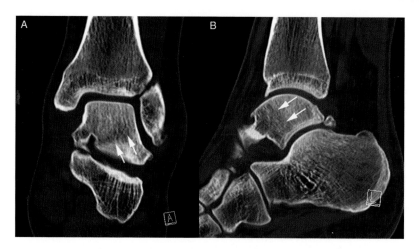

Fig. 7.11 Stress fractures of the ankle can mimic the pain of Achilles tendon rupture. (A, B) Two-dimensional reconstruction computed tomography image showing a vertical radiolucent line *(arrow)* at the lateral region of the talar body. (From Kim YS, Lee HM, Kim JP, et al. Fatigue stress fracture of the talar body: an uncommon cause of ankle pain. *J Foot Ankle Surg.* 2016;55(5):1113-1116 [Fig. 4]. ISSN 1067-2516, https://doi.org/10.1053/j.jfas.2016.01.042, http://www.sciencedirect.com/science/article/pii/S1067251616000430.)

- The patient's symptomatology is the result of an acute injury to the Achilles tendon, although damage and inflammation of the tendon over time may predispose the tendon to rupture.
- Physical examination and testing should focus on identification of causes of the patient's pain and functional disability.
- The patient's pain is localized to the posterior ankle just above the calcaneus.
- Rupture of the proximal Achilles tendon is usually a straightforward clinical diagnosis.
- The patient's symptoms are unilateral and involve only one joint, which is more suggestive of a local process than a systemic polyarthropathy.
- Sleep disturbance is common and must be addressed concurrently with the patient's pain symptomatology.
- Plain radiographs and computerized tomography will provide high-yield information regarding the bony contents of the joint, but ultrasound imaging and MRI will be more useful in identifying soft tissue pathology.
- Although the symptoms of acute rupture of the Achilles tendon appear suddenly, the signs and symptoms of tendinopathy appear more slowly.

Suggested Readings

Al-Saadi S, Michael A. Levofloxacin-induced Achilles tendinitis and tendon rupture. *Eur Geriatr Med*. 2012;3(6):380−381.

Maffulli N, Via AG, Oliva F. Chronic Achilles tendon disorders: tendinopathy and chronic rupture. *Clin Sports Med*. 2015;34(4):607−624.

Malagelada F, Clark C, Dega R. Management of chronic Achilles tendon ruptures—a review. *Foot*. 2016;28:54−60.

Manent A, López L, Coromina H, et al. Acute Achilles tendon ruptures: efficacy of conservative and surgical (percutaneous, open) treatment—a randomized, controlled, clinical trial. *J Foot Ankle Surg*. 2019;58(6):1229−1234.

Moretti L, Solarino G, Pignataro P, et al. Ultrasound and MRI in the assessment of Achilles tendon rupture: are both necessary? *Sports Orthop Traumatol*. 2020;36(4):356−363.

Patel MS, Kadakia AR. Minimally invasive treatments of acute Achilles tendon ruptures. *Foot Ankle Clin*. 2019;24(3):399−424.

Ribbans WJ, Henman PD, Bliss WH. Achilles tendon ruptures in teenagers involved in elite gymnastics. *Sports Orthop Traumatol*. 2016;32(4):375−379.

Tenforde AS, Yin A, Hunt KJ. Foot and ankle injuries in runners. *Phys Med Rehabil Clin N Am*. 2016;27(1):121−137.

Waldman SD. Achilles tendinitis and other abnormalities of the achilles tendon. In: *Waldman's Comprehensive Atlas of Diagnostic Ultrasound of Painful Conditions*. ed. 2. Philadelphia: Wolters Kluwer; 2016:986−996.

Waldman SD, Campbell RSD. Achilles tendon rupture. In: *Imaging of Pain*. ed. 1. Philadelphia: Saunders; 2011:431−432.

Weinfeld SB. Achilles tendon disorders. In: *Med Clin North Am*. 2014;98(2):331−338.

Irina Antipova

A 72-Year-Old Violinist With Right Great Toe Pain

- Learn the common causes of toe pain.
- Develop an understanding of the unique anatomy of the interphalangeal joint of the toes.
- Develop an understanding of the causes of arthritis of the toe.
- Learn the clinical presentation of osteoarthritis of the toe.
- Learn how to use physical examination to identify pathology of the interphalangeal joint of the toes.
- Develop an understanding of the treatment options for osteoarthritis of the interphalangeal joint of the toes.
- Learn the appropriate testing options to help diagnose osteoarthritis of the interphalangeal joint of the toes.
- Learn to identify red flags in patients who present with toe pain.
- Develop an understanding of the role in interventional pain management in the treatment of toe pain.

Irina Antipova

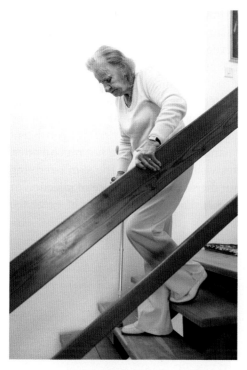

Irina Antipova is a 72-year-old violinist with the chief complaint of, "I can't walk up or down the stairs to my house because of my toe." Irina went on to say that she wouldn't have bothered me, but it was becoming harder and harder to make it up her front steps after coming home from work. Irina said that 50 years of hard winters had finally caught up with her. "Doc, I don't know what I would do if I didn't go to teach my students every day, but the getting up and down the stairs and getting up again is getting harder and harder. I try to use a cane, but it really doesn't help. It takes me forever to get up the stairs. I'm afraid of falling, and my toe hurts so bad."

I asked Irina if anything like this has happened before. She shook her head no, and said that she was in pretty good shape for the shape she was in, but her toes were really hurting, and "walking is getting harder and harder. I never have been a sound sleeper, but that big toe must be waking me up 20 times a night. I have been using my heating pad, but as you know I live alone, and I am afraid to leave it on at night."

I asked Irina about any antecedent trauma to the toes, and she thought about it for a minute. She said that she really couldn't remember any injuries, but back in the "old country," she walked many miles each day and thought nothing of it. "Everyone did, Doc. You worked hard or you starved. The happiest day of my life was when I first laid eyes on the Statue of Liberty."

I asked Irina to point with one finger to show me where it hurt the most. Irina pointed to her right great toe, and then began to rub it. She said, "The whole toe hurts. And the other thing is, sometimes I feel this grating sensation, especially when I first get up in the morning." She denied popping or catching with flexion and extension. I asked if she had any fever or chills, and she shook her head no. "What about steroids?" I asked. "Did you ever take any cortisone or drugs like that?" Irina again shook her head no and said, "Doc, you know me, I'm a tough old bird, and I wouldn't bother you if it didn't really hurt. I love my job—it's my life—but this pain has really got me worried. I have to be able to get up the stairs to get into my house. What will become of me? I am all alone!" And with that, she started crying. I reassured her that we would do all we could to get her better and suggested that we take a look at the toe to figure out what was going on.

On physical examination, Irina was afebrile. Her respirations were 18, and her pulse was 74 and regular. Her blood pressure was normal at 122/74. Her head, eyes, ears, nose, throat (HEENT) exam revealed mild cataract formation on the right. Her cardiopulmonary examination was normal, as was her thyroid exam. Irina's abdominal examination revealed no abnormal mass or organomegaly. There was no costovertebral angle (CVA) tenderness. There was no peripheral edema. Her low back examination was unremarkable. Visual inspection of the toes revealed no cutaneous lesions or deformity other than findings consistent with osteoarthritis. I took a look at her hands and they were not much better, with both Heberden and Bouchard nodes visible (Fig. 8.1). The skin overlying the right great toe was warm to touch, but there was no evidence of infection or rubor that might suggest podogra (Fig. 8.2). Palpation of the right great toe

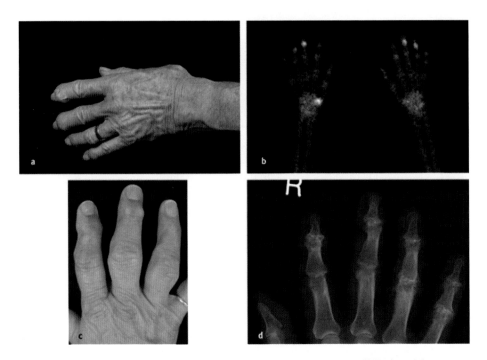

Fig. 8.1 (a) Osteoarthritis of the hand affecting distal interphalangeal joints (DIPJs) and first carpo-metacarpophalangeal (CMC) joint. Note Heberden nodes at DIPJs and squaring at the base of thumb with compensatory hyperextension at the first metacarpophalangeal joint. (b) Bone scan showing increased uptake at DIPJs and first CMC joint. (c) Erosive nodal osteoarthritis with marked joint swelling and deformity. (d) Note classical features of joint space narrowing, sclerosis, and bone cysts on x-ray. Erosions are also present. (From Vincent TL, Watt FE. Osteoarthritis. *Medicine.* 2010;38(3):151–156 [Fig. 2]. ISSN 1357-3039, https://doi.org/10.1016/j.mpmed.2009.11.008, http://www.sciencedirect.com/science/article/pii/S1357303909003454.)

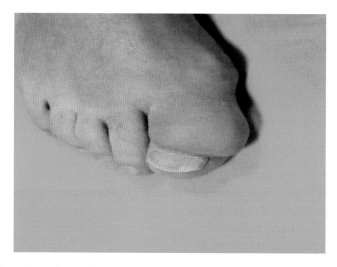

Fig. 8.2 Patient with podogra. Swelling over dorsomedial aspect of first interphalangeal joint of right foot in a patient with acute gouty arthritis. (From Alici T, Imren Y, Erdil M, et al. Gouty arthritis at interphalangeal joint of foot after sildenafil use: a case report. *Int J Surg Case Rep.* 2013;4(1):11–14.)

revealed mild diffuse tenderness, with no obvious synovitis or point tenderness. Range of motion was decreased, with pain exacerbated with active and passive range of motion. The left foot examination was normal, other than findings consistent with osteoarthritis of all the joints of the feet. A careful neurologic examination of the upper and lower extremities revealed no evidence of peripheral or entrapment neuropathy, and the deep tendon reflexes were normal.

Key Clinical Points—What's Important and What's Not

THE HISTORY

- No history of toe trauma
- No fever or chills
- Gradual onset of right great toe pain with exacerbation of pain with use
- Grating sensation in the right toe
- Sleep disturbance
- Difficulty walking up or down stairs due to pain
- Pain on walking

THE PHYSICAL EXAMINATION

- Patient is afebrile
- Normal visual inspection of toe

- Palpation of right great toe reveals diffuse tenderness
- No point tenderness
- Mild warmth of right great toe
- Pain with range of motion
- No evidence of infection
- No active synovitis

OTHER FINDINGS OF NOTE

- Normal blood pressure
- Normal HEENT examination other than mild cataract formation on the right
- Normal cardiovascular examination
- Normal pulmonary examination
- Normal abdominal examination
- No peripheral edema
- No CVA tenderness
- Normal upper extremity neurologic examination, motor and sensory examination

 What Tests Would You Like to Order?

The following tests were ordered:
- Plain radiographs of the right toe

TEST RESULTS

The plain radiographs of the right great toe revealed significant joint space narrowing and osteophyte formation of the first metatarsophalangeal joint consistent with severe osteoarthritis (Fig. 8.3).

 Clinical Correlation—Putting It All Together

What is the diagnosis?
- Osteoarthritis of the right metatarsophalangeal joint of the great right toe

The Science Behind the Diagnosis
ANATOMY OF THE TOE JOINTS

Each toe joint has its own capsule (Fig. 8.4). The articular surface of these joints is covered with hyaline cartilage, which is susceptible to arthritis. The toe joint capsules are lined with a synovial membrane that attaches to the articular cartilage.

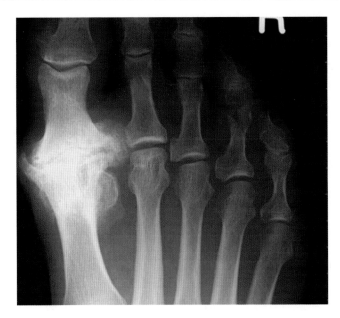

Fig. 8.3 Osteoarthritis of the great toe. Note joint narrowing of the metatarsophalangeal joint of the great toe.

The deep transverse ligaments connect the joints of the five toes and provide the majority of strength to the toe joints. The muscles of the toe joint and their attaching tendons are susceptible to trauma and to wear and tear from overuse and misuse.

CLINICAL CONSIDERATIONS

The toe joint is susceptible to the development of arthritis from various conditions that can damage the joint cartilage. Osteoarthritis is the most common form of arthritis that results in toe joint pain; rheumatoid arthritis and posttraumatic arthritis are also frequent causes of toe pain. Less common causes include the collagen vascular diseases, infection, and Lyme disease. Acute infectious arthritis is usually accompanied by significant systemic symptoms, including fever and malaise, and should be easily recognized; it is treated with culture and antibiotics rather than injection therapy. Collagen vascular disease generally manifests as polyarthropathy rather than as monoarthropathy limited to the toe joint, although toe pain secondary to collagen vascular disease responds exceedingly well to the intraarticular injection technique described later. Gout often affects the first interphalangeal joint of the foot, and the clinical syndrome is known as podogra (Box 8.1; see Fig. 8.2).

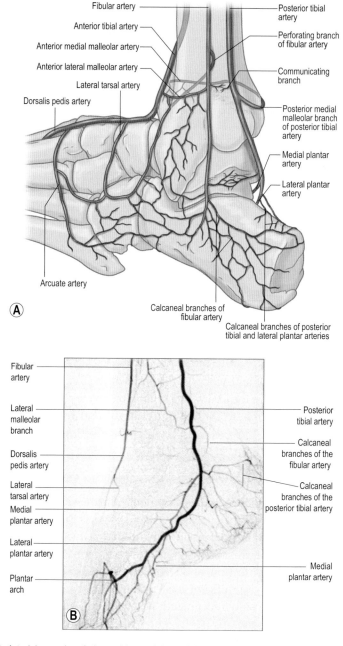

Fig. 8.4 (A) Arterial supply of the ankle and foot. (B) Arteriogram of the ankle and foot. (From Standring S. Gray's, Anatomy: The Anatomic Basis of Clinical Practice. ed. 42. Elsevier; 2021 [Fig. 79-9A].)

BOX 8.1 ■ Risk Factors for Development of Gout

Genetic
- Male sex
- Ancestry
- Genetic markers, including SLC2A9, ABCG2, SLC17A1/SLC17A3, and GCKR

Drugs
- Diuretics
- Cyclosporin
- Tacrolimus
- Angiotensin-converting enzyme inhibitors
- Nonlosartan angiotensin II receptor blockers
- β-blockers
- Pyrazinamide
- Ritonavir

Dietary
- Red meat
- Seafood
- Beer
- Spirits
- Sugar-sweetened beverages

Other
- Increasing age
- Menopause
- Chronic kidney disease
- Overweight, obesity, or weight gain
- Hypertension
- Hyperlipidemia
- Hypertriglyceridemia
- Congestive cardiac failure
- Obstructive sleep apnea
- Anemia
- Psoriasis
- Sickle cell anemia
- Hematologic malignancy
- Lead exposure

Reprinted with permission from Elsevier (from Nicola Dalbeth, Tony R Merriman, Lisa K Stamp. Gout. *The Lancet*. 2016;388(10055):2039–2052 [Fig. 4]. ISSN 0140-6736.)

SIGNS AND SYMPTOMS

Most patients present with pain localized to the affected joint of the foot, most commonly the great toe. Activity, especially flexion of the toe joints, makes the pain worse (Fig. 8.5), whereas rest and heat provide some relief. The pain is constant and is characterized as aching; it may interfere with sleep. Some

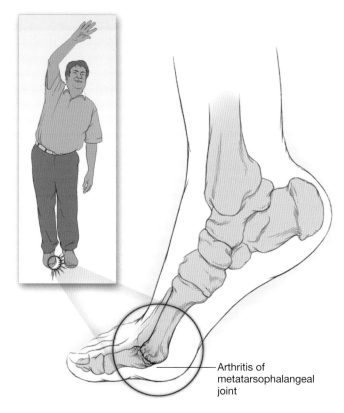

Fig. 8.5 Arthritis of the toe manifests as pain that is made worse with weight-bearing activity. (From Waldman S. *Atlas of Common Pain Syndromes*. ed. 4. Philadelphia: Elsevier; 2019 [Fig. 128-2].)

patients complain of a grating or popping sensation with use of the joint, and crepitus may be present on physical examination. In addition to pain, patients often experience a gradual decrease in functional ability because of reduced toe range of motion that makes simple, everyday tasks such as walking, standing on tiptoes, and climbing stairs quite difficult.

TESTING

Plain radiographs are indicated in all patients who present with toe joint pain (Figs. 8.6 and 8.7; see Figs. 8.1 and 8.3). Magnetic resonance imaging (MRI), computed tomography (CT) scanning, and ultrasound imaging of the toe are indicated if joint instability, an occult mass, or a tumor is suspected (Figs. 8.8, 8.9, 8.10, and 8.11). Based on the patient's clinical presentation, additional testing

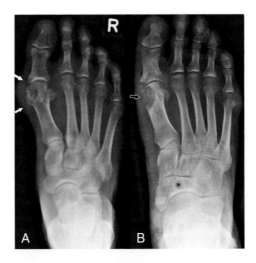

Fig. 8.6 A and B Plain radiograph demonstrating gout involving the right great toe (*white arrows*). (From Dhanda, S, Jagmohan, P, Tian, QS, A re-look at an old disease: A multimodality review on gout. *Clinical Radiology*. 2011;66(10):984—992 [Fig. 1].)

may be warranted, including a complete blood count, erythrocyte sedimentation rate, and antinuclear antibody testing.

DIFFERENTIAL DIAGNOSIS

Bursitis and tendinitis of the foot, as well as entrapment neuropathies such as tarsal tunnel syndrome, may confuse the diagnosis; these conditions may coexist with arthritis of the toes. Gout will often affect the great toe, and acute gouty arthritis of the great toe is known as podogra (see Fig. 8.2). Primary and metastatic tumors of the foot, occult fractures of the tarsals and metatarsals, and fractures of the sesamoid bones of the foot may manifest in a manner similar to arthritis of the toes.

TREATMENT

Initial treatment of the pain and functional disability associated with arthritis of the toes includes a combination of nonsteroidal antiinflammatory drugs or cyclooxygenase-2 inhibitors and physical therapy. The local application of heat and cold may also be beneficial. Avoidance of repetitive activities that aggravate the patient's symptoms, as well as short-term immobilization of the toe joints,

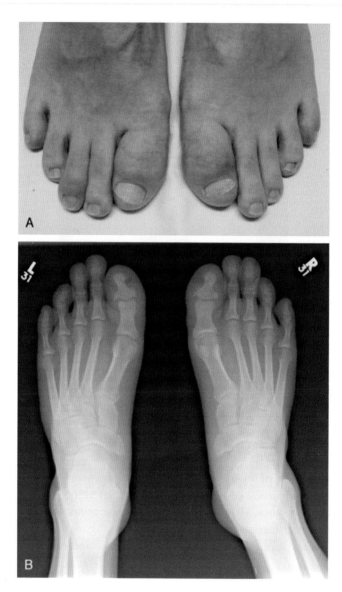

Fig. 8.7   (A) Patient with psoriatic arthritis. Clinical photograph showing dactylitis of both big toes and swelling and redness over the third right toe distal interphalangeal joint. (B) Radiographs of both feet demonstrating erosions and mild periosteal reaction. (From Gladman DD. Management of psoriatic arthritis. In: Weisman MH, Weinblatt ME, Louie JS, et al., eds. *Targeted Treatment of the Rheumatic Diseases*. Philadelphia: Saunders; 2010:55–69.)

may provide relief. For patients who do not respond to these treatment modalities, intraarticular injection with local anesthetic and steroid is a reasonable next step (Fig. 8.12). The injection of platelet-rich plasma and/or stem cells may

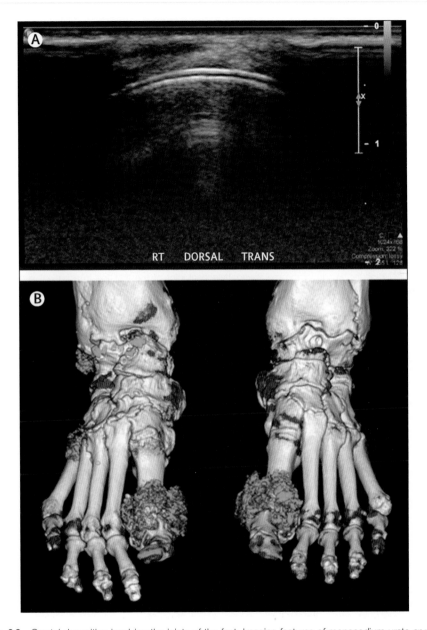

Fig. 8.8 Crystal deposition involving the joints of the feet. Imaging features of monosodium urate crystal deposition. (A) This image shows the double contour sign in the first metatarsophalangeal joint on ultrasonography (tranverse view of the dorsal surface of the joint), defined as hyperechoic enhancement over the surface of the hyaline cartilage. (B) This image shows a dual-energy computed tomography of a patient with tophaceous gout. Urate deposition *(color coded in green)* can be seen at characteristic sites, including the first metatarsophalangeal joint, midfoot, and ankle. Green signal at the nails of the big toes is an artifact commonly observed at this site. Reprinted with permission from Elsevier (from Nicola Dalbeth, Tony R Merriman, Lisa K Stamp. Gout. *The Lancet*. 2016;388(10055):2039–2052 [Fig. 4]. ISSN 0140-6736.)

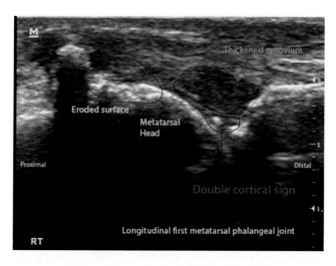

Fig. 8.9 Ultrasound image of the metatarsophalangeal joint of the first toe in a patient with gouty arthritis. Note the double cortical sign, which is highly suggestive for crystal deposition disease.

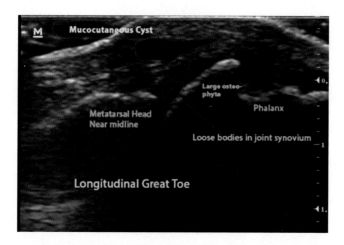

Fig. 8.10 Longitudinal ultrasound image demonstrating joint mice in the metatarsophalangeal joint of the great toe.

reduce the pain and functional disability of arthritis of the toes. Physical modalities, including local heat and gentle range-of-motion exercises, should be introduced several days after the patient undergoes injection. Vigorous exercises should be avoided because they will exacerbate the patient's symptoms.

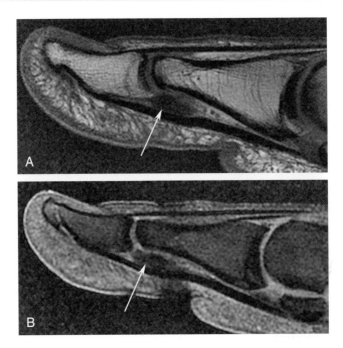

Fig. 8.11 Turf toe. A 23-year-old man with first interphalangeal plantar plate injury. Sagittal T1-weighted (A) and proton density fat suppression (B) images show thickening and indistinctness of the first interphalangeal plantar plate *(arrow).* (From Schein AJ, Skalski MR, Patel DB, et al. Turf toe and sesamoiditis: what the radiologist needs to know. *Clin Imaging.* 2015;39(3):380—389.)

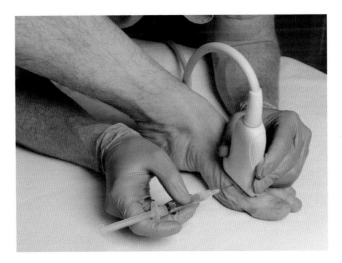

Fig. 8.12 Proper needle position for ultrasound-guided out-of-plane injection of the metatarsophalangeal joint.

HIGH-YIELD TAKEAWAYS

- The patient is afebrile, making an acute infectious etiology (e.g., septic arthritis) unlikely.

- The patient's symptomatology is not the result of acute trauma but more likely the result of repetitive microtrauma that has damaged the joint over time.

- The patient's pain is diffuse rather than highly localized, as would be the case with a pathologic process such as Morton neuroma.

- The patient's symptoms are unilateral and involve only one joint, which is more suggestive of a local process than a systemic polyarthropathy such as polymyalgia rheumatica.

- Sleep disturbance is common and must be addressed concurrently with the patient's pain symptomatology.

- Plain radiographs and CT scanning will provide high-yield information regarding the bony contents of the joint, but ultrasound imaging and MRI will be more useful in identifying soft tissue pathology.

Suggested Readings

Alici T, Imren Y, Erdil M, et al. Gouty arthritis at interphalangeal joint of foot after sildenafil use: a case report. *Int J Surg Case Rep.* 2013;4(1):11–14.

Schein AJ, Skalski MR, Patel DB, et al. Turf toe and sesamoiditis: what the radiologist needs to know. *Clin Imaging.* 2015;39(3):380–389.

Waldman SD. Arthritis and other abnormalities of the metatarsophalangeal and interphalangeal joints. In: *Waldman's Comprehensive Atlas of Diagnostic Ultrasound of Painful Conditions.* ed. 2. Philadelphia: Wolters Kluwer; 2016:1030–1042.

Waldman SD. Arthritis pain of the toe. In: *Atlas of Common Pain Syndromes.* ed. 4. Philadelphia: Elsevier; 2019:507–509.

Waldman SD. Intra-articular injection of the interphalangeal joints of the toes. In: *Atlas of Pain Management Injection Techniques.* ed. 4. Philadelphia: Elsevier; 2017:600–603.

Waldman SD, Campbell RSD. Anatomy: special imaging considerations of the ankle and foot. In: *Imaging of Pain.* ed. 1. Philadelphia: Saunders; 2011:417–420.

Bobby Moltisanti

A 48-Year-Old Meat Cutter With a Painful Bump on His Big Toe

- Learn the common causes of toe pain.
- Learn the common causes of toe deformity.
- Develop an understanding of the anatomy of the toe.
- Develop an understanding of the causes of hallux valgus.
- Develop an understanding of the differential diagnosis of toe pain.
- Learn the clinical presentation of hallux valgus.
- Learn how to use physical examination to identify hallux valgus.
- Develop an understanding of the complications associated with untreated hallux valgus.
- Develop an understanding of the treatment options for hallux valgus.

Bobby Moltisanti

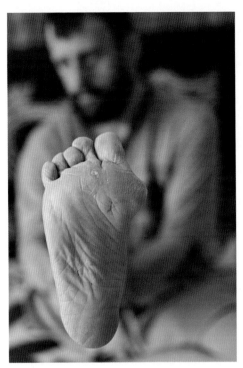

Bobby Moltisanti is a 48-year-old meat cutter with the chief complaint of, "I can't find shoes that will fit because of my big toe." Bobby stated that over the past couple of months, he has been having increasing foot pain. "Doctor, I have ugly feet. My mother, of blessed memory, used to tease me about them. But lately, my feet are killing me. I stand on my feet all day long. It takes a lot of work to cut up those steaks that you and your family like to eat. I thought I needed new shoes, but I bet I tried on 100 pairs and none of them fit. I feel like the bump on my big toe has gotten bigger, and my shoes are just too tight. Doctor, ugly feet I can live with, but my feet hurt all of the time. I go home each day after work and soak my feet in Epsom salts, take some Advil, and go to bed. I don't do anything anymore but watch TV." Bobby went on to say that over the last few months, he began to notice that the bump on the side of his right big toe seemed swollen and a little irritated. "Doc, I've been a meat cutter my whole life. It's all I know, and I can't do it lying in bed. I wish now I had paid a little more attention in school. All I could think about was girls and cars and having fun. Well, let me tell you, I'm not having much fun with this foot pain. I really need to do something about it."

I asked Bobby if he had experienced any numbness or weakness in his feet, and he shook his head and replied, "Never. Doc, the pain is around the bump on my big toe, and it can hurt a bit when I move my toe. I can live with the bump, but the pain is becoming a real problem. I just don't want it to be cancer. If you push on the bump, oh boy! The pain gets a lot worse." I asked Bobby how he was sleeping, and he said, "Not worth a crap, Doc. Every time I roll over, if I move my toes, the pain wakes me up. And the worry about what I'm going to do if I can't work hasn't helped."

I asked Bobby to show me where the pain was, and he pointed to the bump on the side of his great toe (Fig. 9.1)." Doc, the pain is right around this bump." I asked, "Does the pain radiate anywhere?" Bobby shook his head no. "How long has the toe been out of alignment?" I asked Bobby. He replied that it had

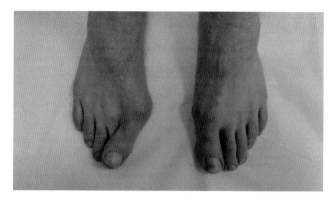

Fig. 9.1 The classic finding of bunion or the hallux valgus deformity. (From Johal S, Sawalha S, Pasapula C. Post-traumatic acute hallux valgus: a case report. *Foot (Edinb)*. 2010;20(2–3):87–89.)

been that way for as long as he could remember, but the pain was something new. "You know, Doc, my mom had the same feet. She spent most of her time in an old pair of house shoes with the part over the bump cut out. I'm working in a freezing cold meat locker, so wearing house shoes is not an option. Besides, do you know what would happen if I dropped a side of beef on my foot if I was wearing house shoes? Not an option." I asked Bobby about any fever, chills, or other constitutional symptoms such as weight loss or night sweats, and he shook his head no. He denied any other joint, musculoskeletal, or systemic symptoms, or bowel or bladder symptoms.

On physical examination, Bobby was afebrile. His respirations were 18, his pulse was 72 and regular, and his blood pressure was 124/76. Bobby's head, eyes, ears, nose, throat (HEENT) exam was normal, as was his thyroid exam. Auscultation of his carotids revealed no bruits, and the pulses in all four extremities were normal. He had a regular rhythm without ectopy. His cardiac exam was otherwise unremarkable. His abdominal examination revealed no abnormal mass or organomegaly. There was no peripheral edema. His low back examination was unremarkable. There was no costovertebral angle (CVA) tenderness. I did a rectal exam, which revealed a completely normal prostate. Visual inspection of the right toe revealed the classic deformity of a bunion: hallux valgus (see Fig. 9.1). There was no evidence of ecchymosis of the skin overlying the bunion. Deep palpation of the bunion elicited pain, as did any effort to straighten the toe. There was no other obvious bony deformity (e.g., hammertoe, which can accompany hallux valgus). The left foot examination was completely normal, as was examination of Bobby's other joints. A careful neurologic examination of both lower extremities was within normal limits. Deep tendon reflexes were physiologic throughout.

Key Clinical Points—What's Important and What's Not

THE HISTORY

- History of right great toe pain and deformity
- The gradual increase in pain in the great toe
- The pain is localized to the great toe and affects no other joints
- Standing can exacerbate the pain
- There is significant sleep disturbance
- No fever or chills

THE PHYSICAL EXAMINATION

- Patient is afebrile
- Classic findings of hallux valgus (bunion) of the right great toe
- Marked tenderness to palpation of the right great toe
- Marked pain with any attempt to straighten deformity of the right great toe
- Normal neurologic examination, specifically no signs of tarsal tunnel syndrome

OTHER FINDINGS OF NOTE

- Normal HEENT examination
- Normal cardiovascular examination
- Normal pulmonary examination
- Normal abdominal examination
- No peripheral edema

 ## What Tests Would You Like to Order?

The following tests were ordered:
- X-ray of the right great toe

TEST RESULTS

X-ray of the toe reveals hallux valgus of the great toe on the right (Fig. 9.2).

 ## Clinical Correlation—Putting It All Together

What is the diagnosis?
- Hallux valgus

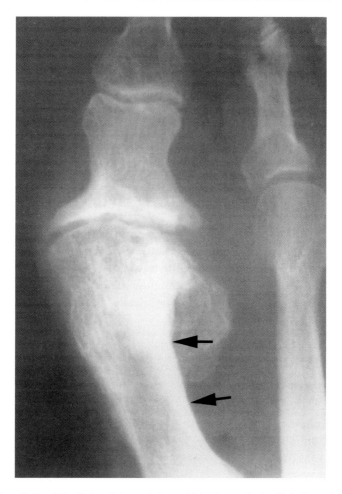

Fig. 9.2 Osteoarthritis of the first metatarsophalangeal joint in a patient with hallux valgus deformity. The sesamoids are lateral to the metatarsal head. The radiograph shows narrowing of the joint space, with subchondral bone and osteophyte formation. Marked thickening of the lateral cortex of the metatarsal shaft *(arrows)* is evident. (From Brower AC, Flemming DJ. *Arthritis in Black and White.* ed. 2. Philadelphia: Saunders; 1997.)

The Science Behind the Diagnosis

ANATOMY

The metatarsophalangeal joints of the toes are condyloid joints characterized by the articulation of the rounded articular surfaces of the metatarsal heads into the shallow concavities of the articular surfaces of the proximal end of the first phalanges (Fig. 9.3). Each joint is lined with synovium, and the ample synovial space allows for intraarticular placement of needles for injection and aspiration. The

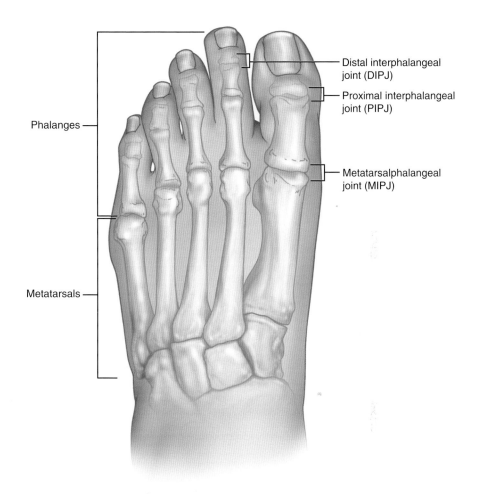

Fig. 9.3 Anatomy of the metatarsophalangeal joint. (From Waldman S. *Atlas of Pain Management Injection Techniques*. ed. 4. St. Louis: Elsevier; 2017 [Fig. 159-2].)

metatarsophalangeal joints have dense joint capsules and strong plantar and collateral ligaments, although fracture and subluxation may still occur. The metatarsophalangeal joints of the toes are also susceptible to overuse and misuse injuries with resultant inflammation and arthritis.

CLINICAL SYNDROME

Bunion, also known as hallux valgus, is one of the most common causes of foot pain. The term *bunion* refers to soft tissue swelling over the first

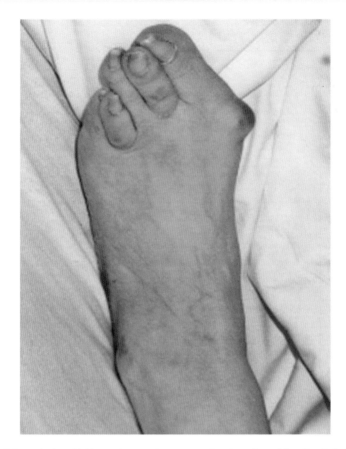

Fig. 9.4 An inflamed adventitial bursa frequently accompanies the pain and functional disability associated with bunion.

metatarsophalangeal joint associated with abnormal angulation of the joint that results in a prominent first metatarsal head and overlapping of the first and second toes, called the hallux valgus deformity. The first metatarsophalangeal joint may ultimately subluxate and cause the overlapping of the first and second toes to worsen (see Fig. 9.1). An inflamed adventitious bursa may accompany bunion formation (Fig. 9.4). The most common cause of bunions is the wearing of narrow-toed shoes, and high heels may exacerbate the problem (Fig. 9.5); thus bunions are more common in women.

SIGNS AND SYMPTOMS

Most patients present with hallux valgus and complain of being unable to find shoes that fit. Walking makes the pain worse, whereas rest and heat provide

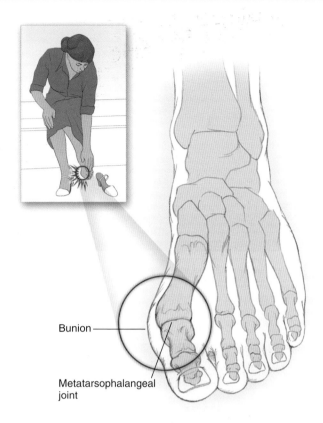

Fig. 9.5   Narrow-toed shoes are implicated in the development of bunions. (From Waldman S. *Atlas of Common Pain Syndromes*. ed. 4. Philadelphia: Elsevier; 2019 [Fig. 129-2].)

some relief. The pain is constant and is characterized as aching; it may interfere with sleep. Some patients complain of a grating or popping sensation with use of the joint, and crepitus may be present on physical examination. In addition to pain, patients with bunions develop the characteristic hallux valgus deformity, with a prominent first metatarsal head, improper angulation of the joint, and overlapping first and second toes (see Fig. 9.1).

TESTING

Plain radiographs are indicated in all patients who present with bunion pain (Fig. 9.6; see Fig. 9.2). Magnetic resonance imaging (MRI), computerized tomography, and ultrasound imaging of the toe are indicated if joint instability, an occult mass, or a tumor is suspected (Figs. 9.7 and 9.8). Based on the patient's

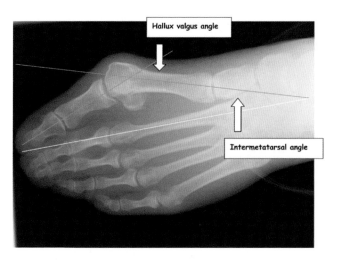

Fig. 9.6 Radiographic assessment of hallux valgus (bunion). (From Thomas S, Barrington R. Hallux valgus. *Curr Orthop*. 2003;17(4):299–307 [Fig. 6]. ISSN 0268-0890, https://doi.org/10.1016/S0268-0890 (02)00184-6, http://www.sciencedirect.com/science/article/pii/S0268089002001846.)

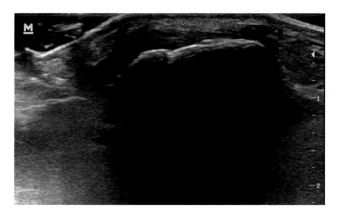

Fig. 9.7 Longitudinal ultrasound view of hallux valgus (bunion). Note the significant adventitial tissue over the lateral great toe. (From Waldman S. *Atlas of Common Pain Syndromes*. ed. 4. Philadelphia: Elsevier; 2019 [Fig. 129-4].)

clinical presentation, additional testing may be warranted, including a complete blood count, erythrocyte sedimentation rate, and antinuclear antibody testing.

DIFFERENTIAL DIAGNOSIS

The diagnosis of bunion is usually obvious on clinical grounds alone. Bursitis and tendinitis of the foot and ankle often coexist with bunion pain. In addition,

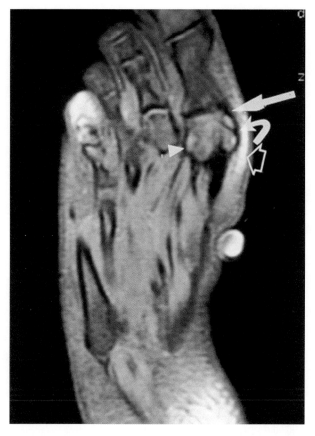

Fig. 9.8   Axial T1-weighted image (488/18) of the foot of a 35-year-old female shows a flat first meta-tarsal head *(arrow)*, a medial eminence *(curved arrow)*, and lateral osteophyte *(arrowhead)*. (From Schweitzer ME, Maheshwari S, Shabshin N. Hallux valgus and hallux rigidus: MRI findings. *Clin Imaging*. 1999;23(6):397−402 [Fig. 4]. ISSN 0899-7071, https://doi.org/10.1016/S0899-7071(00) 00167-4, http://www.sciencedirect.com/science/article/pii/S0899707100001674.)

stress fractures of the metatarsals, phalanges, or sesamoid bones may confuse the diagnosis and require specific treatment. Joplin neuroma, which is perineural fibrosis of the medial plantar digital nerve, is sometimes seen following bunion surgery and may confuse the clinical picture (Fig. 9.9 and Box 9.1).

TREATMENT

Initial treatment of the pain and functional disability associated with bunion includes a combination of nonsteroidal antiinflammatory drugs or cyclooxygenase-2 inhibitors and physical therapy. The local application of heat and cold may also be beneficial. Avoidance of repetitive activities that aggravate the

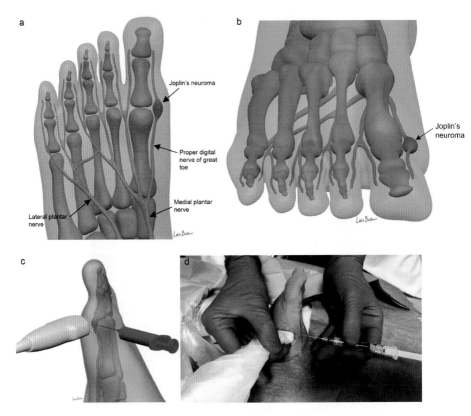

Fig. 9.9 Joplin neuroma. (a—c) Schematic images demonstrating the anatomic course of medial plantar proper digital nerve (MPPDN) of the great toe and associated Joplin neuroma. The MPPDN is the terminal medial branch arising from the medial plantar nerve, passing medially along the hallux where a Joplin neuroma can form. (d) Photograph demonstrating the needle trajectory utilized to inject Joplin nerve. (From Burke CJ, Sanchez J, Walter WR, et al. Ultrasound-guided therapeutic injection and cryoablation of the medial plantar proper digital nerve (Joplin's nerve): sonographic findings, technique, and clinical outcomes. *Acad Radiol.* 2020;27(4):518—527 [Fig. 1]. ISSN 1076-6332, https://doi.org/10.1016/j.acra.2019.05.014, http://www.sciencedirect.com/science/article/pii/S1076633219303046.)

patient's symptoms, avoidance of narrow-toed or high-heeled shoes, and short-term immobilization of the affected toes may also provide relief. For patients who do not respond to these treatment modalities, injection with local anesthetic and steroid is a reasonable next step (Fig. 9.10). Physical modalities, including local heat and gentle range-of-motion exercises, should be introduced several days after the patient undergoes injection. Surgical correction of the hallux valgus deformity may be required for patients who fail to respond to conservative therapy or to correct significant bony deformity.

BOX 9.1 ■ Differential Diagnosis of Hallux Valgus

- Ganglion cyst
- Inflamed bursa
- Synovitis
- Fracture callus
- Exuberant synovium
- Fibroma
- Giant cell tumor
- Aneurysmal bone cyst
- Unicameral bone cyst
- Lipoma
- Neural tumors
- Interosseous ganglions
- Osteoid osteoma
- Osteochondroma
- Osteosarcoma
- Metastatic disease

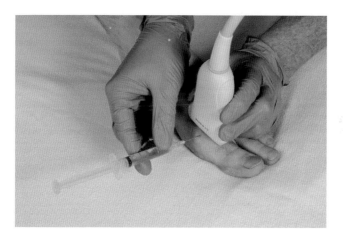

Fig. 9.10 Proper needle position for ultrasound-guided out-of-plane injection of the metatarsophalangeal joint.

HIGH-YIELD TAKEAWAYS

- The patient is afebrile, making an acute infectious etiology unlikely.
- Physical examination and testing should focus on identification of other pathologic processes that may mimic the clinical diagnosis of hallux valgus.

(Continued)

- The patient exhibits physical examination findings that are highly suggestive of hallux valgus.
- The patient's symptoms are localized.
- Plain radiographs of the toe will help identify bony abnormalities of the toe, including fractures, dislocations, and osseous tumors.
- Ultrasound imaging, computerized tomography, and MRI of the toe and pelvis may help identify less common causes of toe pain.

Suggested Readings

Dayton P, Kauwe M, Feilmeier M. Clarification of the anatomic definition of the bunion deformity. *J Foot Ankle Surg*. 2014;53(2):160–163.

Dayton P, Kauwe M, Feilmeier M. Is our current paradigm for evaluation and management of the bunion deformity flawed? A discussion of procedure philosophy relative to anatomy. *J Foot Ankle Surg*. 2015;54(1):102–111.

Mann R. Bunions in the elite athlete: the philosophy and principles. In: Porter DA, Schon LC, eds. *Baxter's The Foot and Ankle in Sport*. ed. 3. Philadelphia: Elsevier; 2021:411–415.

Melendez MM, Patel A, Dellon AL. The diagnosis and treatment of Joplin's neuroma. *J Foot Ankle Surg*. 2016;55(2):320–323.

Waldman SD. Arthritis and other abnormalities of the metatarsophalangeal and interphalangeal joints. In: *Waldman's Comprehensive Atlas of Diagnostic Ultrasound of Painful Conditions*. ed. 2. Philadelphia: Wolters Kluwer; 2016:1030–1042.

Waldman SD. Bunion pain. In: *Atlas of Common Pain Syndromes*. ed. 4. Philadelphia: Elsevier; 2019:510–512.

Waldman SD. Hallux valgus deformity. In: *Waldman's Comprehensive Atlas of Diagnostic Ultrasound of Painful Conditions*. Philadelphia: Wolters Kluwer; 2016:1043–1048.

Waldman SD. Injection technique for bunion pain syndrome. In: *Atlas of Pain Management Injection Techniques*. ed. 4. Philadelphia: Saunders; 2017:661–663.

Miranda Halliday

A 24-Year-Old Fashion Designer With Pain in Her Little Toe

- Learn the common causes of foot pain.
- Develop an understanding of the unique anatomy of the fifth metatarsophalangeal joint.
- Develop an understanding of the causes of bunionette.
- Develop an understanding of the differential diagnosis of bunionette.
- Learn the clinical presentation of bunionette.
- Learn how to examine the foot.
- Learn how to use physical examination to identify bunionette.
- Develop an understanding of the treatment options for bunionette.

Miranda Halliday

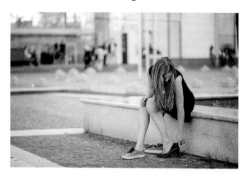

Miranda Halliday is a 24-year-old fashion designer with the chief complaint of, "My left little toe is killing me." Miranda stated that she was traveling to a fashion show in New York about 3 weeks ago when she did something "really stupid." She packed several pairs of new Christian Louboutin high heels that a supplier had given her to wear on the trip. Miranda must have noticed the blank look on my face, and she said, "You know, Doctor, the ones with the red bottoms?" I nodded as convincingly as I could, and said, "So what about these shoes caused your foot pain?" She said, "Doctor, have you ever worn high heels that were a size too small for 15 hours a day? Let me tell you, it's something you really, really, really do not want to do. I should have packed some more comfortable shoes, but I was in a hurry to catch my flight—really, really, really stupid." She called an Uber to take her to her hotel and told the driver to take her to the Hilton, but they took her to the wrong Hilton. "I got to the front desk and they couldn't find my reservation. They called around and saw that I was actually staying at the New York Hilton Midtown, not the Hilton Times Square where the Uber dropped me off. The desk clerk said it was an easy walk, so off I went. Because, as you can see, I am really fit, a 20-block walk seemed like no biggie. I made it about 10 blocks when my left foot really started to hurt. I just figured that my feet had swollen on the plane, and once I put my feet up, I would be fine. I know, I know, I have a bad habit of wearing shoes that are a little small, but who wants a girl with size 9 feet?"

I asked Miranda about any antecedent foot trauma, and she shook her head no, but went on to say that over the last 6 months, she had noticed that her left little toe was looking a little funny. She also noted that she was getting some calluses on the tops of her other toes (Fig. 10.1). When she went to get a pedicure, the girl told her that her shoes were rubbing on the top of her toes, but high heels are a part of her job, her look, her brand narrative. Usually after a couple of Extra-Strength Tylenols and a glass of wine or two, she was good to go. This time, the pain just wouldn't go away. Miranda said she felt that her left little toe was starting to go sideways and asked, "What was that all about?" She said that after a day on her feet, the little toe and the side of her foot were kind of swollen and "squishy," and felt irritated and warm to touch. I asked Miranda what made her pain worse, and she said wearing some pairs of shoes was worse than others, and long days on her feet, like during Fashion Week, were the worst. "Sometimes a heating pad will help, but I really don't like that my little toe is

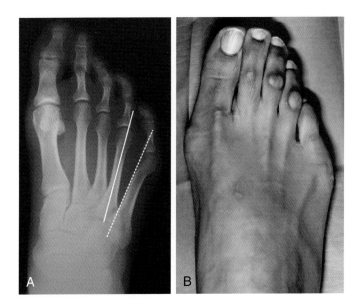

Fig. 10.1   (A) Tailor's bunion deformity may be assessed radiographically with a lateral splaying in the distal fifth metatarsal. (B) Clinically, the patient generally presents with symptoms occurring laterally or plantarlaterally, often with an adduction of the fifth toe. (From Clinical Practice Guideline Forefoot Disorders Panel; Thomas JL, Blitch EL IV, Chaney DM, et al. Diagnosis and treatment of forefoot disorders. IV. Tailor's bunion. *J Foot Ankle Surg.* 2009;48:257–263.)

going all cattywompus on me. Before this, I actually had nice-looking feet. I now have to wear tennis shoes when I walk to work! Doctor, can you believe it?"

I asked Miranda to point with one finger to show me where it hurt the most. She pointed to the lateral aspect of the left little toe and said, "It's really the whole side of my foot that hurts." She cupped the lateral side of her left foot with her right palm for emphasis.

On physical examination, Miranda was afebrile. Her respirations were 18, and her pulse was 64 and regular. Her blood pressure was 119/68. Miranda's head, eyes, ears, nose, throat (HEENT) exam was normal, as was her cardiopulmonary examination. Her thyroid was normal. Her abdominal examination revealed no abnormal mass or organomegaly. There was no costovertebral angle (CVA) tenderness. There was no peripheral edema. Her low back examination was unremarkable. Visual inspection of the left foot revealed findings consistent with a bunionette. There was some swelling over the fifth metatarsophalangeal joint on the left. The toe was warm but did not appear to be infected. The left foot felt slightly edematous on palpation, and there was tenderness over the joint. Palpation of the little toe on the left exacerbated Miranda's pain. Range of motion of the metatarsophalangeal joint also caused an increase in pain. I appreciated some crepitus when I dorsiflexed the toe. The right foot examination was normal, other than some callus formation over the dorsum of the third through fifth toes. Examination of her other major joints revealed no evidence of inflammatory arthropathy. A careful neurologic examination of the lower extremities revealed no evidence of peripheral or entrapment neuropathy, and the deep tendon reflexes were normal.

Key Clinical Points—What's Important and What's Not

THE HISTORY

- History of wearing high heels that were too tight for a long period of time
- No fever or chills
- Swelling of the left little toe
- Deformity of the left little toe

THE PHYSICAL EXAMINATION

- Patient is afebrile
- Medial angulation of the little toe on the left
- Callus formation on the dorsa of the second through fourth toes
- Tenderness to palpation of the left little toe
- Palpation of lateral aspect of the left foot reveals warmth to touch
- Mild swelling in the foot
- No evidence of infection
- Pain on range of motion

OTHER FINDINGS OF NOTE

- Normal HEENT examination
- Normal cardiovascular examination
- Normal pulmonary examination
- Normal abdominal examination
- No peripheral edema
- Normal upper extremity neurologic examination, motor and sensory examination
- Examination of joints other than the left foot were normal other than callus formation on the dorsa of the third through fifth toes on the right

What Tests Would You Like to Order?

The following tests were ordered:
- Plain radiographs of the foot
- Ultrasound of the left foot

TEST RESULTS

The plain radiographs of the left foot lateral splaying of the distal fifth metatarsal are consistent with tailor's bunion (bunionette) (see Fig. 10.1).

 Clinical Correlation—Putting it all Together

What is the diagnosis?
- Bunionette (tailor's bunion)

The Science Behind the Diagnosis

ANATOMY

The metatarsophalangeal joints of the toes are condyloid joints characterized by the articulation of the rounded articular surfaces of the metatarsal heads into the shallow concavities of the articular surfaces of the proximal end of the first phalanges (Fig. 10.2). Each joint is lined with synovium, and the ample synovial space allows for intraarticular placement of needles for injection and aspiration. The metatarsophalangeal joints have dense joint capsules and strong plantar and collateral ligaments, although fracture and subluxation may still occur. The metatarsophalangeal joints of the toes are also susceptible to overuse and misuse injuries with resultant inflammation and arthritis.

CLINICAL SYNDROME

Occurring less commonly than the common bunion, bunionette is a common cause of lateral foot pain. The term *bunionette* refers to a constellation of symptoms, including soft tissue swelling over the fifth metatarsophalangeal joint associated with abnormal angulation of the joint, resulting in a prominent fifth metatarsal head with associated medial angulation (Figs. 10.3 and 10.4). Bunionette also is known as tailor's bunion. This deformity is analogous to the hallux valgus deformity and occurs more commonly in women. The development of an inflamed adventitious bursa may accompany bunionette formation and contribute to the patient's pain. A corn overlying the fifth metatarsal head also is usually present. The most common cause of bunionette formation is the wearing of tight, narrow-toed shoes (Fig. 10.5). High heels may exacerbate the problem.

SIGNS AND SYMPTOMS

Most patients with bunionette complain of pain that is localized to the affected fifth metatarsophalangeal joint and the inability to find shoes that fit. Walking

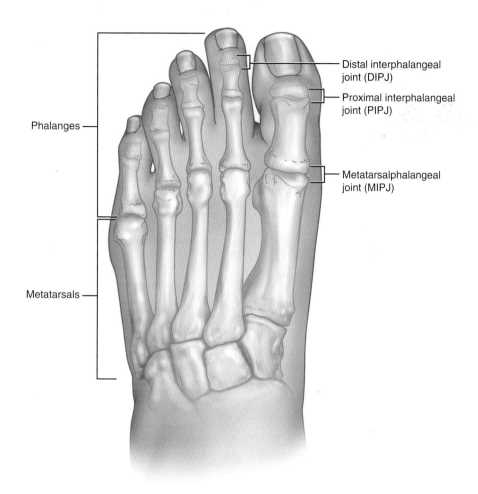

Fig. 10.2 Anatomy of the metatarsophalangeal joint. (From Waldman S. *Atlas of Pain Management Injection Techniques*. ed. 4. St. Louis: Elsevier; 2017 [Fig. 159-2].)

worsens the pain; rest and heat provide some relief. The pain is constant and characterized as aching; it may interfere with sleep. Some patients complain of a grating or popping sensation with use of the joint, and crepitus may be present on physical examination. Physical examination reveals soft tissue swelling over the fifth metatarsophalangeal joint associated with abnormal angulation of the joint, resulting in a prominent fifth metatarsal head with associated medial angulation (Fig. 10.6).

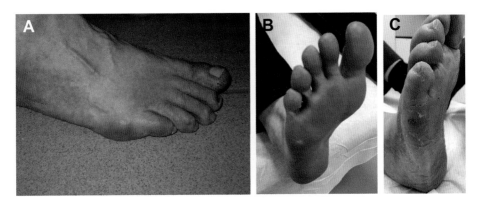

Fig. 10.3 Clinical photographs demonstrating bunionette. Clinical aspects. (A) Painful prominence. (B) Hyperkeratosis. (C) Chronic ulcerations. (From Michels F, Guillo S. Bunionette: is there a minimally invasive solution? *Foot Ankle Clin.* 2020;25(3):425—439 [Fig. 1]. ISSN 1083-7515, ISBN 9780323759090, https://doi.org/10.1016/j.fcl.2020.05.004, http://www.sciencedirect.com/science/article/pii/S1083751520300553.)

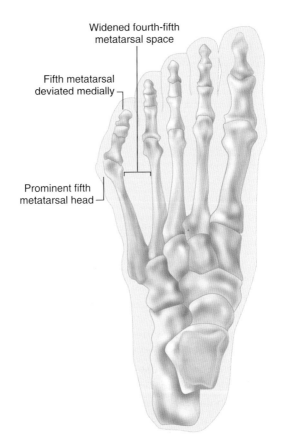

Widened fourth-fifth
metatarsal space

Fifth metatarsal
deviated medially

Prominent fifth
metatarsal head

Fig. 10.4 The bony deformity of bunionette. (From Pfeffer G, Easley M, Hintermann B, et al. *Operative Techniques: Foot and Ankle Surgery.* ed. 2. Philadelphia: Elsevier; 2018 [Fig. 15.3].)

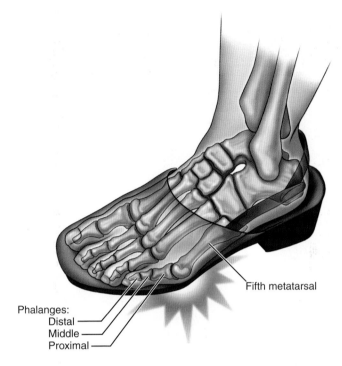

Fifth metatarsal

Phalanges:
Distal
Middle
Proximal

Fig. 10.5 The most common cause of bunionette formation is the wearing of tight, narrow-toed shoes. (From Waldman S. *Atlas of Uncommon Pain Syndromes*. ed. 4. Philadelphia: Saunders; 2020 [Fig. 132-2].)

TESTING

Plain radiographs are indicated in all patients with bunionette pain (Fig. 10.7; see Fig. 10.1). Based on the patient's clinical presentation, additional tests, including complete blood cell count, erythrocyte sedimentation rate, and antinuclear antibody testing, may be indicated. Magnetic resonance imaging (MRI) of the fifth metatarsophalangeal joint is indicated if joint instability, occult mass, or tumor is suspected.

DIFFERENTIAL DIAGNOSIS

The diagnosis of bunionette is usually obvious on clinical grounds alone. Complicating the care of a patient with a typical bunion deformity is the fact that bursitis and tendinitis of the foot and ankle frequently coexist with the bunion pain. Stress fractures of the metatarsals, phalanges, or sesamoid bones also may confuse the clinical diagnosis and require specific treatment.

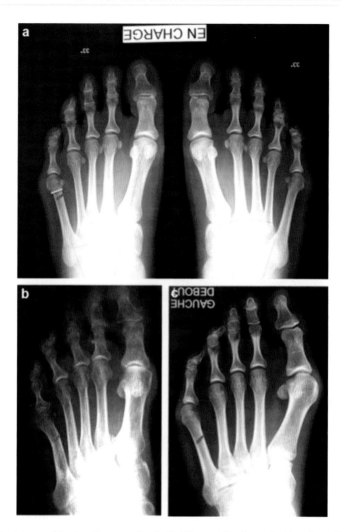

Fig. 10.6 Three types of bunionette according to DuVries and the theoretical location of bone cuts: in red, de Prado medial closing wedge, located in the distal third; in yellow, more distal and complete, allowing a direct translation of the metatarsal head. (a) Type 1 (weight bearing), (b) type 2, (c) type 3 (*left*, standing). (From Laffenêtre O, Millet-Barbe B, Darcel V, et al. Percutaneous bunionette correction: results of a 49-case retrospective study at a mean 34 months' follow-up. *Orthop Traumatol Surg Res.* 2015;101(2):179–184 [Fig. 1].)

TREATMENT

Initial treatment of the pain and functional disability associated with bunionette deformity should include a combination of nonsteroidal antiinflammatory drugs or cyclooxygenase-2 inhibitors and physical therapy. Local application of heat

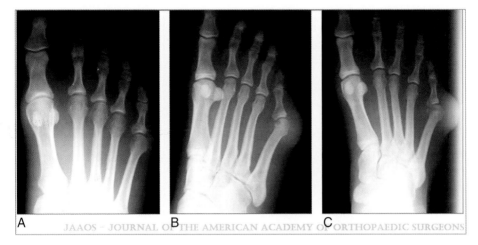

Fig. 10.7 Radiographic classification bunionette deformity. Weight-bearing anteroposterior radiographs demonstrating bunionette classification. (A) Type I, with lateral prominence of the metatarsal head. (B) Type II, with lateral bowing of the fifth metatarsal. (C) Type III, with widening of the 4th to 5th intermetatarsal angle. (From Cohen BE, Nicholson CW. Bunionette deformity. *J Am Acad Orthop Surg*. 2007;15(5):300–307.)

and cold may be beneficial. Avoidance of repetitive activities that aggravate the symptoms and narrow-toed or high-heeled shoes combined with short-term immobilization of the affected toes also may provide relief. For patients who do not respond to these treatment modalities, an injection with a local anesthetic and steroid may be a reasonable next step (Fig. 10.8).

Physical modalities, including local heat and gentle range-of-motion exercises, should be introduced several days after the patient undergoes injection for bunionette. Vigorous exercises should be avoided because they will exacerbate the patient's symptoms. The patient should be cautioned against wearing shoes that are too narrow or too short. Surgical treatment may be required to correct the pain and deformity associated with bunionette in patients who fail to respond to conservative therapy.

HIGH-YIELD TAKEAWAYS

- The patient is afebrile, making an acute infectious etiology (e.g., septic arthritis) unlikely.
- The patient's symptomatology is the result of wearing tight, high-heeled shoes for long periods of time. Physical examination and testing should focus on identification of other ligamentous injury, acute arthritis, tendinitis, and bursitis.

(Continued)

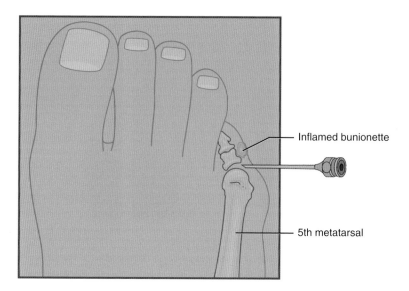

Fig. 10.8 Correct needle placement to inject bunionette. (From Waldman S. *Atlas of Pain Management Injection Techniques*. ed. 4. St. Louis: Elsevier; 2017 [Fig. 176-1].)

- The patient has point tenderness over the deformity of the left little toe, which is highly suggestive of bunionette.
- There is warmth and swelling of the affected joint, suggestive of an inflammatory process.
- The patient's symptoms are unilateral and involve only one joint, which is more suggestive of a local process than a systemic polyarthropathy.
- Plain radiographs will provide high-yield information regarding the bony contents of the joint, but ultrasound imaging and MRI will be more useful in identifying soft tissue pathology.

Suggested Readings

Bertrand T, Parekh SG. Bunionette deformity: etiology, nonsurgical management, and lateral exostectomy. *Foot Ankle Clin*. 2011;16(4):679−688.

DiDomenico L, Baze E, Gatalyak N. Revisiting the tailor's bunion and adductovarus deformity of the fifth digit. *Clin Podiatr Med Surg*. 2013;30(3):397−422.

Laffenêtre O, Millet-Barbé B, Darcel V, et al. Percutaneous bunionette correction: results of a 49-case retrospective study at a mean 34 months' follow-up. *Orthop Traumatol Surg Res*. 2015;101(2):179−184.

Papaliodis DN, Vanushkina MA, Richardson NG, et al. The foot and ankle examination. *Med Clin North Am*. 2014;98(2):181−204.

Redfern DJ, Vernois J. Percutaneous surgery for metatarsalgia and the lesser toes. *Foot Ankle Clin*. 2016;21(3):527–550.

Waldman SD. Arthritis and other abnormalities of the metatarsophalangeal and interphalangeal joints. In: *Waldman's Comprehensive Atlas of Diagnostic Ultrasound of Painful Conditions*. ed. 2. Philadelphia: Wolters Kluwer; 2016:1030–1042.

Waldman SD. Bunionette pain. In: *Atlas of Uncommon Pain Syndromes*. ed. 4. Philadelphia: Elsevier; 2021:447–448.

Waldman SD. Injection technique for bunion pain syndrome. In: *Atlas of Pain Management Injection Techniques*. ed. 4. Philadelphia: Saunders; 2017:661–663.

Sarah Davidow

A 64-Year-Old Homemaker With Foot Pain

- Learn the common causes of foot pain.
- Develop an understanding of the unique anatomy of the digital nerves.
- Develop an understanding of the causes of Morton neuroma.
- Develop an understanding of the differential diagnosis of Morton neuroma.
- Learn the clinical presentation of Morton neuroma.
- Learn how to examine the foot.
- Learn how to use physical examination to identify Morton neuroma.
- Develop an understanding of the treatment options for Morton neuroma.

Sarah Davidow

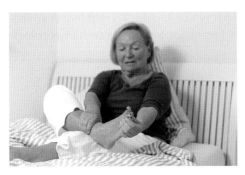

Sarah Davidow is a 64-year-old homemaker with the chief complaint of, "I feel like I'm walking on a stone." Sarah stated that over the past several months, her right foot started "hurting when I walked. I kept taking my shoe off and dumping it out because I thought something was in it, but nothing was there." She went on to say, "This is so embarrassing. My husband, Artie, says it's all in my head." I asked Sarah if she had ever had anything like this before, and she said, "Absolutely not. I have beautiful feet, and they have never bothered me. I get a pedicure every couple of weeks, and lately it hurts when the gal pushes the pressure points on the bottom of my feet."

I asked Sarah what made her foot pain worse, and she said that whenever she put any weight on her right foot, she felt the stone. It was really bad when she stood on the tile floor of her kitchen for any length of time. "Doctor, I used to take Lucky, that's my Yorkie, on long walks, but I just can't do it anymore. Lucky and I are both putting on weight! Doctor, you don't think this is cancer or something bad, do you? It just won't get better!"

I asked her what made the pain better, and she said Advil seemed to help a little but not with the "stone in the shoe" sensation. Advil, however, upset her stomach. She noted that the heating pad felt good, but she thought it made her foot swell. "I also tried using an Ace wrap, but I felt like it was cutting off my circulation." I asked Sarah about any antecedent foot trauma, and she could not recall anything.

I asked Sarah to point with one finger to show me where it hurt the most. She pointed to the ball of her foot and said, "Right here." I told her that I had a pretty good idea what was going on, and we would do all we could to get it fixed.

On physical examination, Sarah was afebrile. Her respirations were 16, and her pulse was 74 and regular. Her blood pressure was 126/76. Sarah's head, eyes, ears, nose, throat (HEENT) exam was normal, as was her cardiopulmonary examination. Her thyroid was normal. Her abdominal examination revealed no abnormal mass or organomegaly. There was no costovertebral angle (CVA) tenderness. There was no peripheral edema. Her low back examination revealed some tenderness to deep palpation of the paraspinous musculature. Visual inspection of the right foot revealed no bony abnormality or evidence of a plantar wart. The Tinel sign over the deep peroneal nerve was negative bilaterally, and Sarah had no numbness between the web of her great and second toes, decreasing the probability of anterior tarsal tunnel syndrome. The Mulder sign was positive on the right, as was the digital nerve stretch test. Both were negative on the left (Figs. 11.1 and 11.2). Range of motion of the foot joint, especially resisted extension and passive flexion of the foot joint, caused Sarah to cry out in pain. The left foot examination was normal, as was examination of her major joints. A careful neurologic

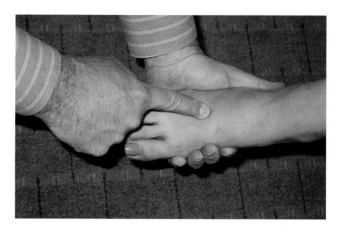

Fig. 11.1 Eliciting Mulder sign for Morton neuroma. Mulder sign is elicited by firmly squeezing the metatarsal heads together with one hand while placing firm pressure on the interdigital space with the other. (From Waldman SD. *Physical Diagnosis of Pain: An Atlas of Signs and Symptoms*. Philadelphia: Saunders; 2006:381.)

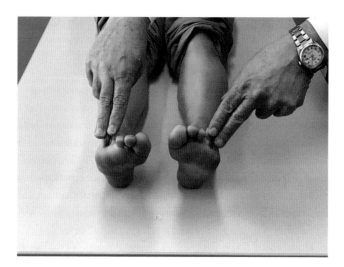

Fig. 11.2 To perform the digital nerve stretch test for Morton neuroma, the patient is placed in the supine position. The patient is then asked to bring both ankles into full dorsiflexion. The examiner then fully extends the toes on each side of the webspace suspected of harboring the Morton neuroma. The test is positive if this maneuver reproduces the patient's symptoms.

examination of the upper and lower extremities revealed no evidence of peripheral or entrapment neuropathy, and the deep tendon reflexes were normal.

Key Clinical Points—What's Important and What's Not

THE HISTORY

- Gradual onset of pain in the ball of the patient's foot
- Patient complaint that it felt like walking on a stone
- Pain made worse with weight bearing and walking
- No other specific traumatic event to the area identified
- No fever or chills

THE PHYSICAL EXAMINATION

- Patient is afebrile
- Pain with palpation of the plantar interdigital space
- Positive Mulder sign
- Positive digital nerve stretch test
- No evidence of infection

OHER FINDINGS OF NOTE

- Normal HEENT examination
- Normal cardiovascular examination
- Normal pulmonary examination
- Normal abdominal examination
- No tenderness to deep palpation of the lumbar paraspinous muscles
- No peripheral edema
- Normal upper and lower extremity neurologic examination, motor and sensory examination
- Examination of joints other than the right foot was normal

 ## What Tests Would You Like to Order?

The following tests were ordered:
- Ultrasound of the left foot

TEST RESULTS

Ultrasound examination of the left foot revealed a large Morton neuroma between the second and third metatarsals (Fig. 11.3).

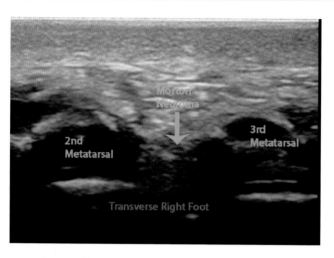

Fig. 11.3 Transverse ultrasound image demonstrating a large Morton neuroma between the second and third metatarsals. (From Waldman S. *Atlas of Common Pain Syndromes*. ed. 4. Philadelphia: Elsevier; 2019 [Fig. 130-5].)

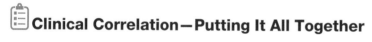 Clinical Correlation—Putting It All Together

What is the diagnosis?

■ Morton neuroma

The Science Behind the Diagnosis

ANATOMY

In a manner analogous to that of the digital nerves of the hand, the digital nerves of the foot travel through the intrametatarsal space to innervate each toe. The plantar digital nerves, which are derived from the posterior tibial nerve, provide sensory innervation to the major portion of the plantar surface (Fig. 11.4). These nerves are subject to entrapment and resultant development of perineural fibrosis and degeneration, resulting in the clinical syndrome known as Morton neuroma (Fig. 11.5). The dorsal aspect of the foot is innervated by terminal branches of the deep and superficial peroneal nerves. The overlap of the innervation of these nerves may be considerable.

CLINICAL SYNDROME

Morton neuroma is one of the most common pain syndromes affecting the forefoot. It is characterized by tenderness and burning pain in the plantar

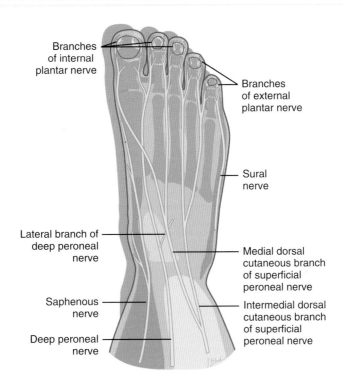

Fig. 11.4 The digital nerves of the foot. (From Waldman S. *Atlas of Interventional Pain Management*. ed. 5. Philadelphia: Elsevier; 2021 [Fig. 155.1].)

surface of the forefoot, with painful paresthesias in the two affected toes. This pain syndrome is thought to be caused by perineural fibrosis of the interdigital nerves (Fig. 11.6). Although the nerves between the third and fourth toes are affected most commonly, the second and third toes and, rarely, the fourth and fifth toes can be affected as well (Fig. 11.7). Patients may feel like they are walking with a stone in the shoe. The pain of Morton neuroma worsens with prolonged standing or walking for long distances and is exacerbated by poorly fitting or improperly padded shoes. As with bunion and hammer toe deformities, Morton neuroma is associated with wearing tight, narrow-toed shoes.

SIGNS AND SYMPTOMS

On physical examination, pain can be reproduced by performing the Mulder maneuver: firmly squeezing the two metatarsal heads together with one hand while placing firm pressure on the interdigital space with the other (see Fig. 11.1).

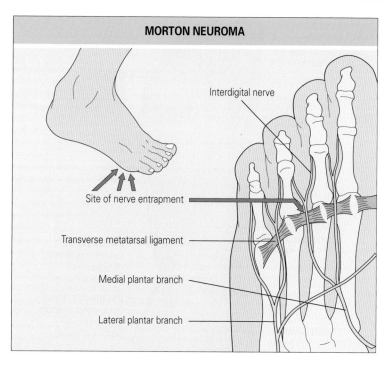

Fig. 11.5 The plantar digital nerves, which are derived from the posterior tibial nerve, provide sensory innervation to the major portion of the plantar surface. These nerves are subject to entrapment and resultant development of perineural fibrosis and degeneration, resulting in the clinical syndrome known as Morton neuroma. (From Hochberg M, Silman A, Smolen J, et al. *Rheumatology*. ed. 6. St. Louis: Mosby; 2015 [Fig. 81-15].)

In contrast to metatarsalgia, in which the tender area is over the metatarsal heads, with Morton neuroma, the tender area is localized to only the plantar surface of the affected interspace, with paresthesias radiating into the two affected toes. Patients suffering from Morton neuroma will exhibit a digital nerve stretch test (see Fig. 11.2). Patients may also exhibit a positive Tinel sign when the interdigital nerve is percussed from the plantar surface of the affected foot. Patients with Morton neuroma often exhibit an antalgic gait in an effort to reduce weight bearing during walking.

TESTING

Plain radiographs, ultrasound imaging, and magnetic resonance imaging (MRI) are indicated in all patients who present with Morton neuroma to rule out fractures and to identify sesamoid bones that may have become inflamed (Fig. 11.8;

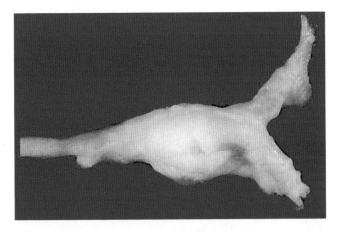

Fig. 11.6 Morton neuroma. Gross photograph of a segment of the plantar interdigital nerve resected from the space between the third and fourth metatarsal heads in a patient with Morton neuroma shows fusiform swelling of the neurovascular bundle just proximal to the bifurcation. (From Benign soft tissue tumors. In: Bullough PG, ed. *Orthopaedic Pathology*. ed. 5. Philadelphia: Mosby; 2010:497–532.)

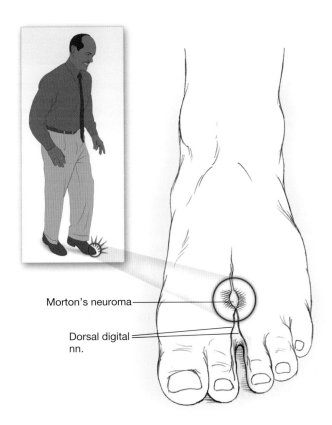

Morton's neuroma

Dorsal digital nn.

Fig. 11.7 The pain of Morton neuroma is made worse with prolonged standing or walking. The patient suffering from Morton neuroma will often complains that it feels like walking on a stone. (From Waldman S. *Atlas of Common Pain Syndromes*. ed. 4. Philadelphia: Elsevier; 2019 [Fig. 130-2].)

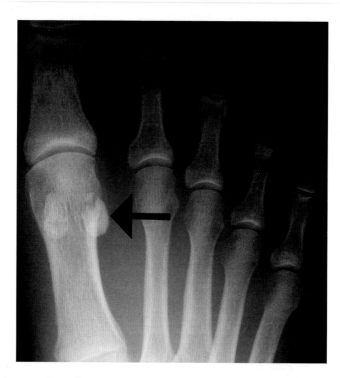

Fig. 11.8 Anteroposterior radiographic view demonstrating irregular shape and sclerosis of the fibular sesamoid *(arrow)*. (From Williams G, Kenyon P, Fischer B, et al. An atypical presentation of hallucial sesamoid avascular necrosis: a case report. *J Foot Ankle Surg.* 2009;48(2):203–207 [Fig. 1]. ISSN 1067-2516, https://doi.org/10.1053/j.jfas.2008.11.004, http://www.sciencedirect.com/science/article/pii/S1067251608004535.)

see Fig. 11.3). Computer tomography scanning may help identify occult bony abnormalities not seen on plan radiographs or other imaging modalities. MRI of the metatarsal bones is also indicated if joint instability, an occult mass, or a tumor is suspected. Ultrasound imaging may also aid in the diagnosis of Morton neuroma (Fig. 11.9). Radionuclide bone scanning may be useful to identify stress fractures of the calcaneus, metatarsal, phalanges, or sesamoid bones that may be missed on plain radiographs (Fig. 11.10). Based on the patient's clinical presentation, additional testing may be warranted, including a complete blood count, erythrocyte sedimentation rate, and antinuclear antibody testing.

DIFFERENTIAL DIAGNOSIS

Fractures of the sesamoid bones of the foot are often confused with Morton neuroma; although the pain of sesamoid fracture is localized to the plantar surface of

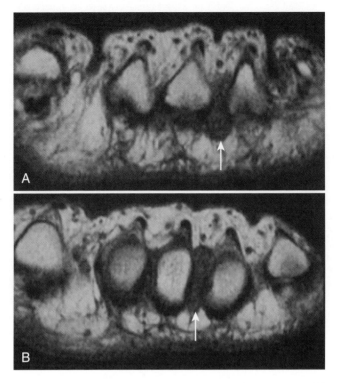

Fig. 11.9 (A, B) Magnetic resonance imaging of Morton neuroma (Arrows indicate Morton neuroma). (From Waldman SD, Campbell RS. *Imaging of Pain*. Elsevier; 2011.)

the foot, it is less neuritic than that of Morton neuroma (Fig. 11.11). Tendinitis, bursitis, and stress fractures of the foot can also mimic the pain of Morton neuroma.

TREATMENT

Initial treatment of the pain and functional disability associated with Morton neuroma includes a combination of nonsteroidal antiinflammatory drugs or cyclooxygenase-2 inhibitors and physical therapy. The local application of heat and cold may also be beneficial. Avoidance of repetitive activities that aggravate the patient's symptoms, avoidance of narrow-toed or high-heeled shoes, and short-term immobilization of the affected foot may also provide relief. For patients who do not respond to these treatment modalities, injection with local anesthetic and steroid is a reasonable next step (Fig. 11.12). Surgical extirpation of the Morton neuroma may be required for patients who fail to respond to more conservative measures (Fig. 11.13).

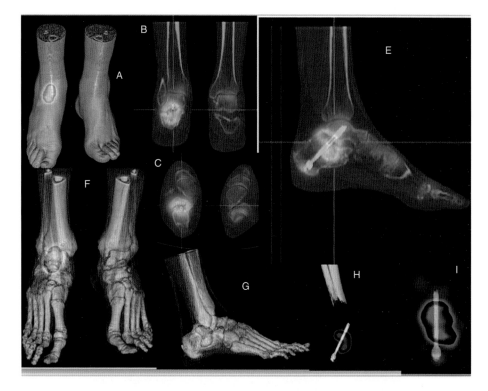

Fig. 11.10 Scintigraphy with disphosphonates labeled with 99mTc. (A, F–I) Three-dimensional reconstruction of volume with different grades of opacity. (B–E) Coronal, axial, and sagittal reconstructions of the single-photon emission computed tomography (SPECT)/computed tomography (CT). A 48-year-old male with a history of right foot pain secondary to a calcaneal fracture. Hardware from a previous surgery is noted. (From Jiménez RG, García-Gómez FJ, Álvarez EN, et al. Hybrid imaging in foot and ankle disorders. *Rev Española Med Nuclear Imag Molecul (English Ed).* 2018;37(3):191–202 [Fig. 3]. ISSN 2253-8089, https://doi.org/10.1016/j.remnie.2017.11.021, http://www.sciencedirect.com/science/article/pii/S225380891730191X.)

A. Distal pole fracture

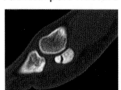

B. Central fragmentation

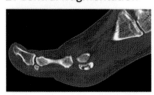

C. Wide separation of fracture fragments

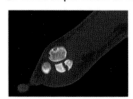

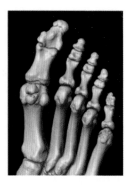

D. 3-D reconstruction of tibial sesamoid stress fracture

Fig. 11.11 (A-D) Computed tomography imaging of sesamoid fractures. (From Ribbans WJ, Hintermann B. Hallucal sesamoid fractures in athletes: diagnosis and treatment. *Sport Orthop Traumatol.* 2016;32(3):295–303 [Fig. 3]. ISSN 0949-328X, https://doi.org/10.1016/j.orthtr.2016.04.001, http://www.sciencedirect.com/science/article/pii/S0949328X16300291.)

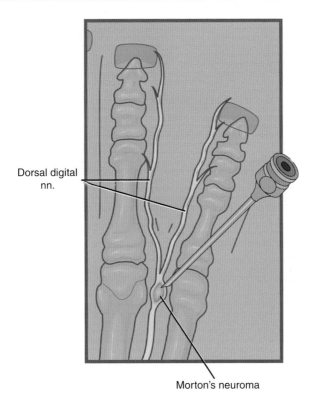

Dorsal digital
nn.

Morton's neuroma

Fig. 11.12 Proper needle placement for injection of Morton neuroma. (From Waldman SD. *Atlas of Pain Management Injection Techniques*. Philadelphia: Saunders; 2000.)

HIGH-YIELD TAKEAWAYS

- The patient is afebrile, making an acute infectious etiology (e.g., septic arthritis) unlikely.
- The patient's symptomatology is highly suggestive of Morton neuroma; physical examination and testing should focus on the identification of ligamentous injury, acute arthritis, tendinitis, and bursitis that may also be contributing to the patient's pain symptomatology.
- The patient's symptoms are unilateral and involve only one joint, which is more suggestive of a local process than a systemic polyarthropathy.
- Ultrasound imaging is highly specific in the diagnosis of Morton neuroma.
- Plain radiographs and computed tomography scanning will provide high-yield information regarding the bony contents of the foot and the identification of fractures or other bony abnormalities of the femur as well as calcification of the bursa and tendons.
- Ultrasound imaging and MRI will be more useful in identifying soft tissue pathology that may be mimicking the clinical presentation of Morton neuroma.

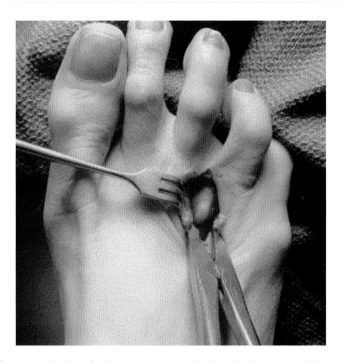

Fig. 11.13 Surgical extirpation of a Morton neuroma using the dorsal approach. Note the large neuroma in situ. (From Singh SK, Ioli JP, Chiodo CP. The surgical treatment of Morton's neuroma. *Curr Orthop.* 2005;19(5):379–384 [Fig. 2]. ISSN 0268-0890, https://doi.org/10.1016/j.cuor.2005.07.004, http://www.sciencedirect.com/science/article/pii/S0268089005001271.)

Suggested Readings

Bhatia M, Thomson L. Morton's neuroma—current concepts review. *J Clin Orthop Trauma.* 2020;11(3):406–409.

Richardson DR, Dean EM. The recurrent Morton neuroma: what now? *Foot Ankle Clin.* 2014;19(3):437–449.

Waldman SD. Injection technique for Morton neuroma syndrome. In: *Atlas of Pain Management Injection Techniques.* ed. 4. Philadelphia: Elsevier; 2017:670–673.

Waldman SD. Morton neuroma syndrome. In: *Waldman's Comprehensive Atlas of Diagnostic Ultrasound of Painful Conditions.* Philadelphia: Wolters Kluwer; 2016: 1063–1070.

Waldman SD, Campbell RSD. Anatomy: special imaging considerations of the ankle and foot. In: *Imaging of Pain.* Philadelphia: Saunders; 2011:417–420.

Waldman SD, Campbell RSD. Morton neuroma. In: *Imaging of Pain.* Philadelphia: Saunders; 2011:459–460.

Ross Marquette

A 68-Year-Old Retired Executive With Severe Posterior Foot Pain

- Learn the common causes of foot pain.
- Learn the common causes of plantar fasciitis.
- Develop an understanding of the anatomy of the plantar fascia.
- Develop an understanding of the differential diagnosis of plantar fasciitis.
- Learn the clinical presentation of plantar fasciitis.
- Learn how to examine the foot.
- Learn how to examine the plantar fascia.
- Learn how to use physical examination to identify plantar fasciitis.
- Develop an understanding of the treatment options for plantar fasciitis.

Ross Marquette

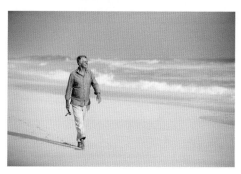

Ross Marquette is a 68-year-old retired executive with the chief complaint of, "I can't exercise because my feet are killing me." Ross stated that over the last 6 weeks, his right foot has become increasingly more painful in spite of Advil, topical analgesic balm, and ice packs. He stated that since he retired and moved to the beach, he was "falling apart." He stated, "My friends told me not to retire, and I should have listened to them, but you know, I had done all there was to do and the buyout offer was just too good to turn down. I have a place on the beach in Hilton Head, and it seemed like the perfect place to get my life back. I wanted to get in shape and started walking on the beach every day, rain or shine. I get up and head down to the beach, no meetings, no employees, no aggravation. Now I feel like somebody is stabbing me in the bottom of my feet! Mostly on the right, but now the left heel is starting to play up. It's worse when I first get up—those first few steps are murder." Ross tried to "work through it" because he didn't want to "mess with his routine." He noted that the pain was made worse with prolonged standing, and it was getting to where walking on the beach was just too painful. "Doctor, I didn't retire to sit on my butt and watch the Golf Channel. I really hope that you can help me here."

I asked Ross if he ever had anything like this in the past, and he said, "Not really. I always tried to watch my weight, but I spent most of the last 35 years sitting at a desk." I asked if he was experiencing any numbness, and he shook his head no. "But you know, Doc, the craziest thing is, when I wiggle my toes, I get a sharp pain in the soles of my feet. It's really painful. I've started walking like an old man." I asked Ross about any fever, chills, or other constitutional symptoms such as weight loss or night sweats, and he shook his head no, and said, "It's just this foot pain. I just don't understand how walking barefoot down a sandy beach could hurt so much!"

I then asked Ross to point with one finger to show me where it hurt the most. He pointed to his right foot and then gingerly rubbed the sole of his right foot up toward his toes and said that the pain seemed to shoot from the heel up toward his toes.

On physical examination, Ross was afebrile. His respirations were 16, his pulse was 66 and regular, and his blood pressure was 112/68. Ross's head, eyes, ears, nose, throat (HEENT) exam was normal, as was his cardiopulmonary examination. His thyroid was normal and his neck was well muscled. His abdominal examination revealed no abnormal mass or organomegaly. There was no

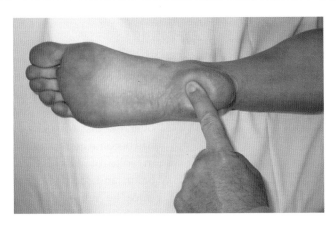

Fig. 12.1 To elicit the calcaneal jump sign, the patient is placed in a supine position on the examination table. The examiner uses the index finger to firmly press on the skin overlying the plantar medial calcaneal tuberosity. The calcaneal jump sign is considered positive if this maneuver reproduces the patient's pain and causes the patient to jump or withdraw from the sudden onset of pain. (From Waldman SD. *Physical Diagnosis of Pain: An Atlas of Signs and Symptoms*. Philadelphia: Saunders; 2006:379.)

costovertebral angle (CVA) tenderness. There was no peripheral edema. His low back examination was unremarkable. I noticed that he was wearing flip-flops. Visual inspection of the right foot was unremarkable. There was no rubor and no obvious infection. There was no evidence of a plantar wart, fibromatosis, or obvious bony abnormality. There was no evidence of Achilles tendonitis or bursitis. Palpation of the sole of the foot along the plantar fascia from the heel to the toe reproduced Ross's pain, as did active resisted dorsiflexion of the toes. Ross had positive calcaneal jump signs bilaterally, right greater than left (Fig. 12.1). The windlass test was also positive bilaterally, again right greater than left (Fig. 12.2). The calcaneal squeeze test for calcaneal stress fracture was negative bilaterally (Fig. 12.3). The left foot examination was normal. A careful neurologic examination of the lower extremities was completely normal, with no evidence of entrapment or peripheral neuropathy. Deep tendon reflexes were normal.

Key Clinical Points—What's Important and What's Not

THE HISTORY

- History of onset of right heel pain associated with walking barefoot on the beach
- No numbness
- No weakness
- No history of previous significant foot pain
- No fever or chills

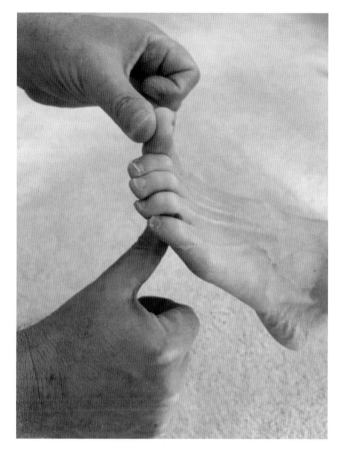

Fig. 12.2   The windlass test for plantar fasciitis. To perform the windlass test for plantar fasciitis, the patient is placed in the supine position with the knee flexed to 90 degrees and the affected foot in neutral position. The examiner then stabilizes the head of the first metatarsal and dorsiflexes the great toe. The test is positive if it reproduces or exacerbates the patient's pain.

THE PHYSICAL EXAMINATION

- Patient is afebrile
- Point tenderness over plantar aspect of the calcaneus
- Pain on active resisted dorsiflexion of the toes
- Pain on palpation of the plantar fascia
- Positive calcaneal jump sign—right greater than left
- Positive windlass sign—right greater than left
- Negative calcaneal squeeze test
- No plantar masses

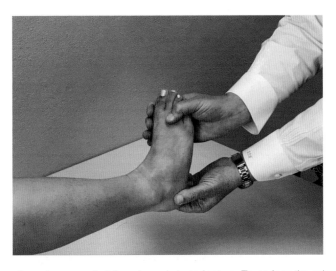

Fig. 12.3   The calcaneal squeeze test for calcaneal stress fracture. To perform the calcaneal squeeze test, the patient is placed in the sitting position in the middle of the examination table with the legs resting comfortably off the side of the table. The examiner holds the affected foot with one hand and grasps the painful calcaneus and gently squeezes, gradually applying greater pressure. The test is considered positive if the pressure reproduces the patient's pain. (From Waldman S. *Physical Diagnosis of Pain: An Atlas of Signs and Symptoms*. ed. 4. Philadelphia: Elsevier; 2021 [Fig. 276-1].)

OTHER FINDINGS OF NOTE

- Normal HEENT examination
- Normal cardiovascular examination
- Normal pulmonary examination
- Normal abdominal examination
- No peripheral edema
- Normal lower extremity neurologic examination, motor and sensory examination

What Tests Would You Like to Order?

The following tests were ordered:
- Plain radiographs of the right foot
- Ultrasound of the right foot
- Magnetic resonance imaging (MRI) of the right foot

TEST RESULTS

The plain radiographs of the right foot revealed a plantar spur on the calcaneus (Fig. 12.4).

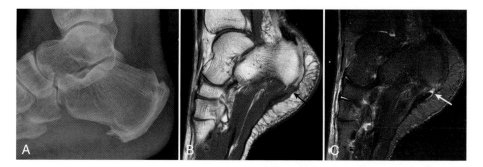

Fig. 12.4 (A) Lateral radiograph of a plantar spur on the calcaneus. (B) The sagittal T1-weighted (T1W) magnetic resonance imaging (MRI) demonstrates thickening and increased signal intensity (SI) within the plantar fascia origin *(black arrow)*. There is high-SI fatty marrow within the bony spur. (C) High-SI fluid *(white arrow)* is seen within the plantar fascia origin on the sagittal fat-suppressed T2W MRI. The appearances are consistent with plantar fasciitis and partial tearing of the origin of the fascia. (From Waldman RS, Campbell RSD. *Imaging of Pain*. Philadelphia: Elsevier; 2011.)

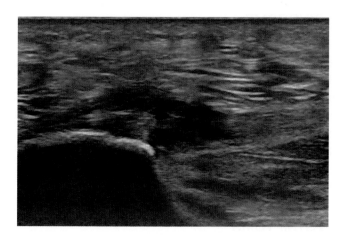

Fig. 12.5 Longitudinal ultrasound image demonstrating a partial tear of the plantar fascia near its insertion on the calcaneus.

Ultrasound examination of the right foot revealed partial tearing of the plantar fascia (Fig. 12.5).

MRI scan of the right foot revealed a partial tear at the origin of the plantar fascia as well as thickening of the plantar fascia consistent with plantar fasciitis (see Fig. 12.4).

Clinical Correlation—Putting It All Together

What is the diagnosis?

- Plantar fasciitis
- Partial tear of the plantar fascia

The Science Behind the Diagnosis

ANATOMY

The plantar fascia is made up of thick, longitudinally oriented connective tissue that is tightly attached to the plantar skin (Fig. 12.6). It attaches to the medial calcaneal tuberosity and then runs forward, dividing into five bands, one going to each toe (Fig. 12.7). The plantar fascia provides dynamic support to the arch of the foot, tightening as the foot bears weight.

CLINICAL SYNDROME

Plantar fasciitis is characterized by pain and tenderness over the plantar surface of the calcaneus. It is twice as common in women as in men. Plantar fasciitis is thought to be caused by inflammation of the plantar fascia, which can occur alone or as part of a systemic inflammatory condition such as rheumatoid arthritis, Reiter syndrome, or gout. Obesity seems to predispose patients to the development of plantar fasciitis, as does going barefoot or wearing house slippers for prolonged periods (Fig. 12.8). High-impact aerobic exercise has also been implicated as a causative factor.

SIGNS AND SYMPTOMS

The pain of plantar fasciitis is most severe when first walking after a period of non-weight bearing and is made worse by prolonged standing or walking. On physical examination, patients exhibit a positive calcaneal jump sign, which consists of point tenderness over the plantar medial calcaneal tuberosity (see Fig. 12.1). The patient may also exhibit a positive windlass test (see Fig. 12.2). Patients may also have tenderness along the plantar fascia as it moves anteriorly. Pain is increased by dorsiflexing the toes, which pulls the plantar fascia taut, and then palpating along the fascia from the heel to the forefoot.

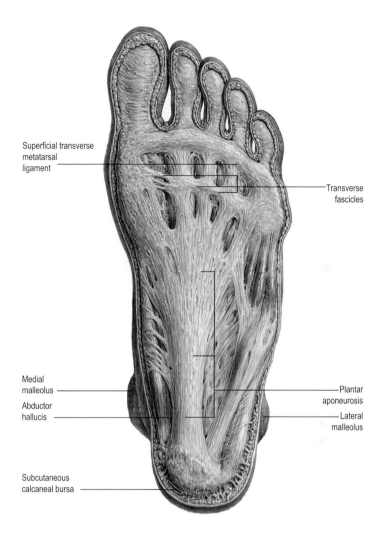

Fig. 12.6 The anatomy of the plantar fascia. (Paulsen, Waschke. *Sobotta Atlas of Human Anatomy.* ed. 16. 2018 © Elsevier GmbH, Urban & Fischer, Munich.)

TESTING

Plain radiographs, MRI, and ultrasound imaging are indicated in all patients who present with pain thought to be caused by plantar fasciitis to rule out occult bony disorders and tumor (Figs. 12.9, 12.10, and 12.11). Although characteristic radiographic changes are lacking in plantar fasciitis, ultrasound imaging will routinely demonstrate thickening of the plantar fascia (Figs. 12.12 and 12.13). Radionuclide bone scanning may show increased uptake where the plantar

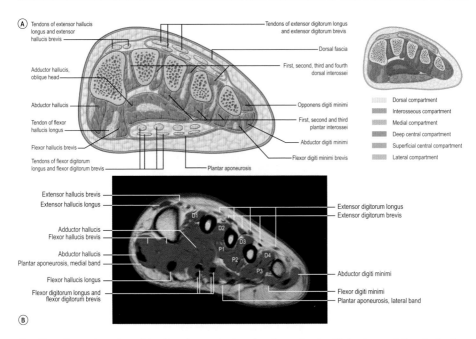

Fig. 12.7 Coronal section of the foot demonstrating the plantar fascia. (A) Anatomy of the plantar fascia. (B) MRI demonstrating the plantar fascia and related structures. (From Standring S. *Gray's Anatomy: The Anatomic Basis of Clinical Practice*. ed. 42. Philadelphia: Elsevier; 2021 [Fig. 79-4].)

fascia attaches to the medial calcaneal tuberosity; it can also rule out stress fractures not visible on plain radiographs. Based on the patient's clinical presentation, additional testing may be warranted, including a complete blood count, prostate-specific antigen level, erythrocyte sedimentation rate, and antinuclear antibody testing. The injection technique described later serves as both a diagnostic and a therapeutic maneuver.

DIFFERENTIAL DIAGNOSIS

Common causes of heel pain are listed in Box 12.1. The pain of plantar fasciitis may be confused with many diseases, including the pain of Sever disease, Morton neuroma, plantar fibromatosis, inclusion cysts, or sesamoiditis (Figs. 12.14 and 12.15). However, the characteristic pain on dorsiflexion of the toes associated with plantar fasciitis should help distinguish these conditions. Stress fractures of the metatarsal or sesamoid bones, bursitis, and tendonitis may also confuse the clinical picture. Complete rupture of the plantar fascia will present with the acute onset of pain, swelling, and ecchymosis of the plantar surface (Figs. 12.16 and 12.17).

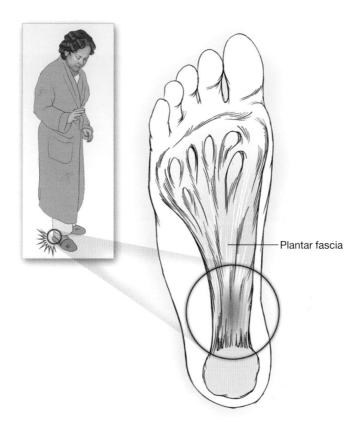

Plantar fascia

Fig. 12.8 The pain of plantar fasciitis, which is localized to the hindfoot, can cause significant functional disability. Obesity seems to predispose patients to the development of plantar fasciitis, as does going barefoot or wearing house slippers for prolonged periods. High-impact aerobic exercise has also been implicated as a causative factor. (From Waldman S. *Atlas of Common Pain Syndromes.* ed. 4. Philadelphia: Elsevier; 2019 [Fig. 133-1].)

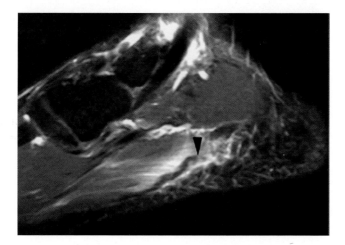

Fig. 12.9 Rupture of the central cord of the plantar fascia. This sagittal short tau inversion recovery magnetic resonance image demonstrates discontinuity of the plantar fascia, with extensive edema of the flexor digitorum brevis muscle *(arrowhead)*. (From Edelman RR, Hesselink JR, Zlatkin MB, et al., eds. *Clinical Magnetic Resonance Imaging.* ed. 3. Philadelphia: Saunders; 2006:3456.)

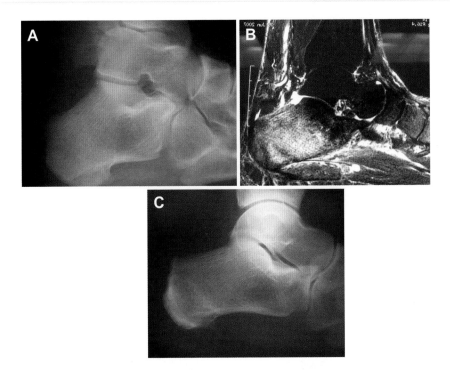

Fig. 12.10 (A) Runner with plantar heel pain. X-ray taken at day 5 of pain is negative. (B) T2-weighted magnetic resonance imaging showing a calcaneal stress fracture. (C) X-ray finally became positive for a calcaneal stress fracture at week 4. (From Toomey EP. Plantar heel pain. *Foot Ankle Clin.* 2009;14 (2):229–245 [Fig. 5]. ISSN 1083-7515, https://doi.org/10.1016/j.fcl.2009.02.001, http://www.science-direct.com/science/article/pii/S1083751509000175.)

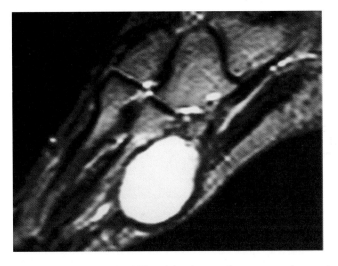

Fig. 12.11 Synovial sarcoma. This sagittal T2-weighted magnetic resonance image demonstrates a large soft tissue mass in the plantar aspect of the foot. The mass is homogeneous and exhibits a thick capsule, simulating a fluid collection. (From Edelman RR, Hesselink JR, Zlatkin MB, et al., eds. *Clinical Magnetic Resonance Imaging.* ed. 3. Philadelphia: Saunders; 2006:3456.)

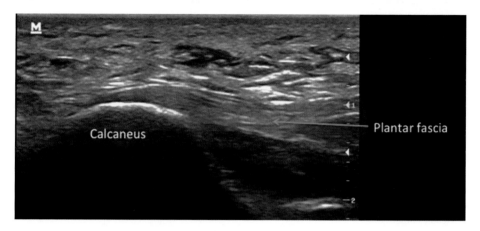

Fig. 12.12 Longitudinal view of the normal plantar fascia and its calcaneal insertion. Note the homogeneous fibular pattern and normal thickness.

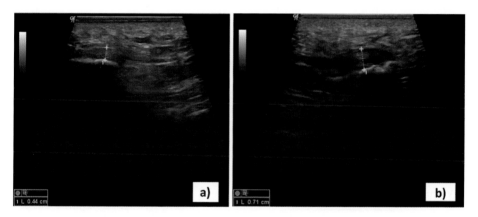

Fig. 12.13 Ultrasound imaging in B-mode demonstrating mild (a) and marked (b) degrees of plantar fascia thickening (measuring 4.4 and 7.1 mm in thickness, respectively) in two different patients in this study. Note the inhomogenicity of the thickened fascia with scattered hypoechoic areas within its substance (more manifest in b). (From Baz AA, Gad AM, Waly MR. Ultrasound guided injection of platelet rich plasma in cases of chronic plantar fasciitis. *Egypt J Radiol Nuclear Med*. 2017;48(1):125–132 [Fig. 1]. ISSN 0378-603X, https://doi.org/10.1016/j.ejrnm.2016.12.004, http://www.sciencedirect.com/science/article/pii/S0378603X16302339.)

TREATMENT

Initial treatment of the pain and functional disability associated with plantar fasciitis includes a combination of nonsteroidal antiinflammatory drugs (NSAIDs) or cyclooxygenase-2 inhibitors and physical therapy. The local application of

BOX 12.1 ■ Differential Diagnosis of Heel Pain

Skeletal

Calcaneal stress fracture
Tarsal stress fractures
Subtalar arthritis
Sever disease
Psoriatic arthritis
Reiter syndrome
Infections, osteomyelitis
Inflammatory arthropathies (e.g., Reiter syndrome, psoriatic arthritis)

Soft Tissue

Achilles tendonitis
Heel pad contusion
Achilles tendon rupture
Retrocalcaneal bursitis
Achilles bursitis
Posterior tibialis tendonitis
Fat pad atrophy
Plantar fascia rupture

Neurologic

Tarsal tunnel syndrome
Lumbar radiculopathy
Entrapment of injury of the medial calcaneal branch of the posterior tibial nerve
Peripheral neuropathies
Abductor digiti quinti nerve entrapment

Miscellaneous

Neuromas
Gout
Crystal arthropathies
Tumors
Metabolic disorders
Osteomalacia
Paget disease
Sickle cell disease
Vascular insufficiency

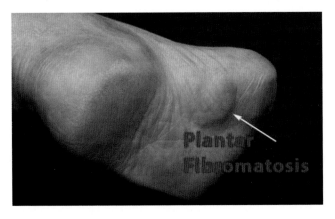

Fig. 12.14 Typical nodule of plantar fibromatosis. Note medial location.

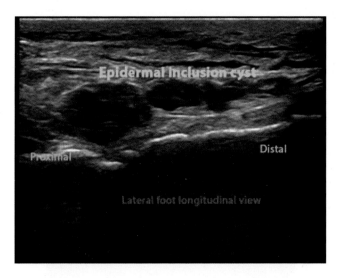

Fig. 12.15 Longitudinal ultrasound image of the plantar surface demonstrating an epidermoid inclusion cyst.

heat and cold may also be beneficial. Avoidance of repetitive activities that aggravate the patient's symptoms, avoidance of walking barefoot or with shoes that do not provide good support, and short-term immobilization of the affected foot may provide relief. For patients who do not respond to these treatment modalities, injection with local anesthetic and steroid is a reasonable next step (Fig. 12.18). Physical modalities, including local heat and gentle stretching exercises, should be introduced several days after the patient undergoes injection. Vigorous exercises should be avoided because they will exacerbate the patient's symptoms. Stretching exercises may be of particular benefit (Fig. 12.19). Heel pads or molded orthotic devices may also be of value. Low-energy extracorporeal shockwave therapy may also provide symptomatic relief in resistant cases. Simple analgesics, NSAIDs, and antimyotonic agents, such as tizanidine, can be used concurrently with this injection technique.

HIGH-YIELD TAKEAWAYS

- The patient is afebrile, making an acute infectious etiology unlikely.
- The patient's symptomatology is consistent with the classic presentation of plantar fasciitis.
- Walking barefoot or in flip-flops or slippers is a common inciting event.

(Continued)

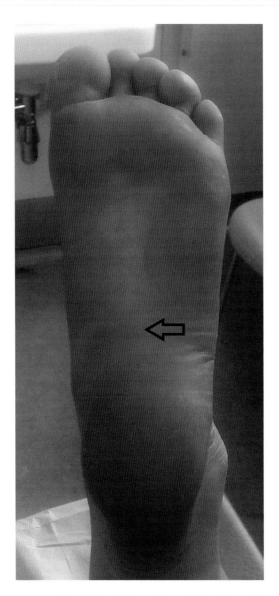

Fig. 12.16 Clinical appearance after plantar fascia rupture with bruising and swelling *(arrow)*. (From Schaarup SO, Burgaard P, Johannsen FE. Surgical repair of complete plantar fascia ruptures in high-demand power athletes: an alternative treatment option. *J Foot Ankle Surg*. 2020;59(1):195–200 [Fig. 1]. ISSN 1067-2516, https://doi.org/10.1053/j.jfas.2019.07.018, http://www.sciencedirect.com/science/article/pii/S106725161930256X.)

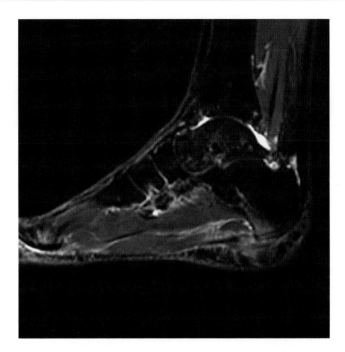

Fig. 12.17 Magnetic resonance imaging showing rupture of the plantar fascia. (From Schaarup SO, Burgaard P, Johannsen FE. Surgical repair of complete plantar fascia ruptures in high-demand power athletes: an alternative treatment option. *J Foot Ankle Surg.* 2020;59(1):195–200 [Fig. 2]. ISSN 1067-2516, https://doi.org/10.1053/j.jfas.2019.07.018, http://www.sciencedirect.com/science/article/pii/S106725161930256X.)

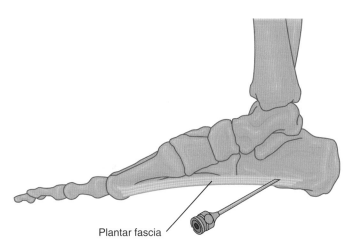

Plantar fascia

Fig. 12.18 Proper needle placement for injection of the calcaneal insertion of the planter fascia. (From Waldman S. *Atlas of Pain Management Injection Techniques.* ed. 4. St. Louis: Elsevier; 2017 [Fig. 171-5].)

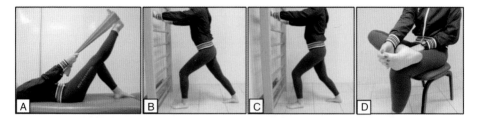

Fig. 12.19   Stretching exercises for plantar fasciitis. (A) Straight leg raise in supine position. (B) Plantar flexor muscles stretch with knee extended. (C) Plantar flexor muscles stretch with knee flexed. (D) Plantar fascia stretch. (From Kamonseki AH, Gonçalves GA, Yi LC, et al. Effect of stretching with and without muscle strengthening exercises for the foot and hip in patients with plantar fasciitis: a randomized controlled single-blind clinical trial. *Manual Therapy*. 2016;23:76–82.)

- Physical examination and testing should focus on identification of other diseases that may mimic the clinical presentation of plantar fasciitis.
- The patient exhibits physical examination findings that are highly suggestive of plantar fasciitis.
- The patient's symptoms are unilateral, which is more suggestive of a local process than a systemic inflammatory process.
- Plain radiographs will provide high-yield information regarding the bony contents of the foot and ankle, but ultrasound imaging and MRI will be more useful in identifying soft tissue pathology that may be responsible for plantar fasciitis.

Suggested Readings

Gogna P, Gaba S, Mukhopadhyay R, et al. Plantar fasciitis: a randomized comparative study of platelet rich plasma and low dose radiation in sportspersons. *Foot (Edinb)*. 2016;28:16–19.

Huffer D, Hing W, Newton R, et al. Strength training for plantar fasciitis and the intrinsic foot musculature: a systematic review. *Phys Ther Sport*. 2017;24:44–52.

Rose B, Singh D. Inferior heel pain. *Orthop Trauma*. 2016;30(1):18–23.

Waldman SD. Injection technique for plantar fasciitis. In: *Atlas of Pain Management Injection Techniques*. ed. 4. Philadelphia: Elsevier; 2017:648–651.

Waldman SD. Plantar fasciitis. In: *Pain Review*. ed. 2. Philadelphia: Elsevier; 2017: 314–315.

Waldman SD. Plantar fasciitis and other abnormalities of the plantar fascia. In: *Waldman's Comprehensive Atlas of Diagnostic Ultrasound of Painful Conditions*. Philadelphia: Wolters Kluwer; 2016:1005–1019.

Waldman SD, Campbell RSD. Plantar fasciitis. In: *Imaging of Pain*. Philadelphia: Saunders; 2011:457–458.

CHAPTER

13

Ada Hunt

A 31-Year-Old Customer Service Representative With Pain in the Arch of the Left Foot

LEARNING OBJECTIVES

- Learn the common causes of foot pain.
- Develop an understanding of the innervation of the groin and pelvis.
- Develop an understanding of the anatomy of the posterior tibial tendons.
- Develop an understanding of the causes of posterior tibial tendinitis.
- Learn the clinical presentation of posterior tibial tendinitis.
- Learn how to use physical examination to identify posterior tibial tendinitis.
- Develop an understanding of the treatment options for posterior tibial tendinitis.
- Learn the appropriate testing options to help diagnose posterior tibial tendinitis.
- Learn to identify red flags in patients who present with foot pain.
- Develop an understanding of the role in interventional pain management in the treatment of posterior tibial tendinitis.

Ada Hunt

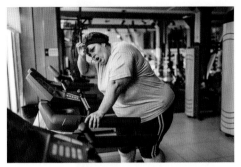

Ada Hunt is a 31-year-old customer service representative with the chief complaint of, "I pulled something in my foot, so I can't exercise." She explained to me, "Doctor, I have to exercise if I'm ever going to lose this weight. And I was doing so well! I've already lost 40 pounds. I just have to exercise, or I am dead." Ada went on to say that since the weather got cold, she had been running on a treadmill rather than outside. The pain came on gradually, but it is so bad that it now hurts to bear any weight on her left foot. "Doctor, I got a new pair of running shoes, but that didn't help. What am I going to do? I'm really having a hard time getting better in spite of massage, acupuncture, aromatherapy, Motrin, and a lidocaine patch." She said she took a few pain pills that she had left over from having her wisdom teeth pulled, but they seized up her bowels, so she quit taking them, too.

I asked Ada if she ever had anything like this before, and she shook her head no. She also denied any current urinary or gynecologic symptoms, hematuria, or fever or chills. She also denied a history of previous foot or ankle injuries. Her last menstrual period was about 10 days ago. Ada is using oral contraceptives. I asked what she was currently doing to manage the pain, and she said, "Nothing really works—the Motrin barely takes the edge off." I asked her to rate her pain on a scale of 1 to 10, with 10 being the worst pain she ever had. She said the pain was a 7 or 8. "Doctor, I have to get back to normal. I have to exercise. The pain is interfering with just about everything. I can't walk, I can't run, I can't do aerobics. I am having a hard time getting around. I just really need to get my life back."

I asked Ada to point with one finger to show me where it hurt the most. She pointed to the medial longitudinal arch of her foot, and said, "Doc, the pain is right here, right under the bone. It's really killing me."

On physical examination, Ada was afebrile. Her respirations were 16. Her pulse was 72 and regular, and her blood pressure was normal at 118/68. Her weight was 276 pounds. Her head, eyes, ears, nose, throat (HEENT) exam was normal, as was her thyroid examination. Her cardiopulmonary examination was negative. Her abdominal examination revealed no abnormal mass or organomegaly, and no groin mass or hernia was identified. There was no costovertebral angle (CVA) tenderness. There was no peripheral edema. Her low back examination was unremarkable. Her lower extremity neurologic examination was completely normal, with no evidence of tarsal tunnel syndrome. There was point tenderness over the medial longitudinal arch on the left. Active resisted

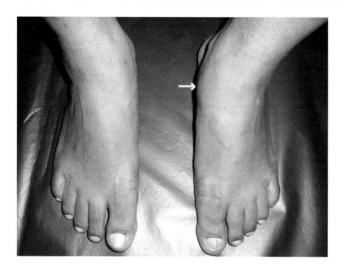

Fig. 13.1   Photograph showing swelling overlying the medial malleolus and the proximal foot with erythema. (From Jakhere SG, Yadav D, Bharambay HV. Acute calcific tendinitis of tibialis posterior tendon (TPT): a rare site of involvement. *Eur J Radiol Extra.* 2011;77(1):e17–e20 [Fig. 1]. ISSN 1571-4675, https://doi.org/10.1016/j.ejrex.2010.10.006, http://www.sciencedirect.com/science/article/pii/S1571467510000799.)

inversion of the ankle reproduced the pain, as did passively flexing the left foot. Visual inspection of the arch revealed no ecchymosis or fibromatosis, but swelling and erythema was noted (Fig. 13.1). "Ada, how about walking down the hall for me?" She carefully sat up and slid off the exam table. As she took off down the hall, I immediately noticed that she had an antalgic gait and was avoiding weight bearing on the left foot.

Key Clinical Points—What's Important and What's Not

THE HISTORY

- History of recent onset of left foot pain following jogging on a treadmill
- Difficulty in ambulating because of left foot pain
- Difficulty in carrying out activities of daily living
- Pain is localized to the medial longitudinal arch of the left foot

THE PHYSICAL EXAMINATION

- Patient is afebrile
- Normal visual inspection of the arch of the left foot
- Tenderness to palpation of the medial longitudinal arch of the left foot

- Active resisted inversion of the left ankle elicits pain
- Passive flexion of the left ankle elicits pain
- Patient has cautious gait with guarding of the left foot with weight bearing
- The lower extremity neurologic examination is within normal limits with no evidence of tarsal tunnel syndrome

OTHER FINDINGS OF NOTE

- Normal blood pressure
- Normal HEENT examination
- Increased body mass index
- Normal cardiopulmonary examination
- Normal abdominal examination
- No peripheral edema
- No groin mass or inguinal hernia
- No CVA tenderness

 ## What Tests Would You Like to Order?

The following tests were ordered:
- X-ray of the left foot
- Ultrasound of the foot with special attention to the posterior tibial tendon
- Magnetic resonance imaging (MRI) of the pelvis with special attention to the posterior tibial tendon

TEST RESULTS

Plain radiograph of the left foot revealed calcific tendinitis of the posterior tibial tendon with no evidence of fracture or other bony abnormality (Fig. 13.2).

Ultrasound imaging reveals acute tendinitis of the posterior tibial tendon with a significant effusion (Fig. 13.3).

MRI with contrast reveals subtle enhancement in the thickened tibialis posterior tendon consistent with posterior tibial tendinitis (Fig. 13.4).

 ## Clinical Correlation—Putting It All Together

What is the diagnosis?
- Posterior tibial tendinitis

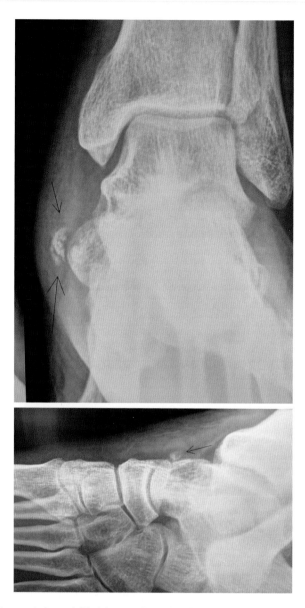

Fig. 13.2   (A) Anteroposterior and (B) oblique radiographs of the ankle showing an area of amorphous, fluffy, irregular calcification adjacent to the medial border of navicular bone. (From Jakhere SG, Yadav D, Bharambay HV. Acute calcific tendinitis of tibialis posterior tendon (TPT): a rare site of involvement. *Eur J Radiol.* 2011;77(1):e17–e20 [Figs. 2, 3]. ISSN 1571-4675, https://doi.org/10.1016/j.ejrex.2010.10.006, http://www.sciencedirect.com/science/article/pii/S1571467510000799.)

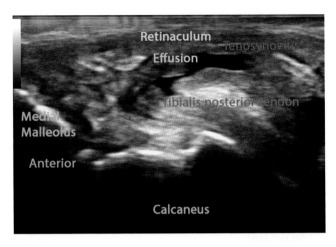

Fig. 13.3   Ultrasound image demonstrating acute tenonsynovitis of the posterior tibial tendon. Note the significant effusion.

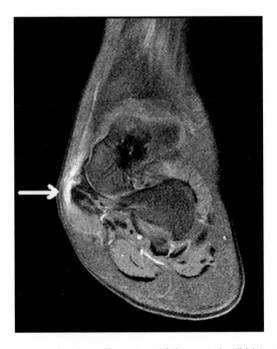

Fig. 13.4   Magnetic resonance imaging with contrast of the posterior tibial tendon. Postgadolinium coronal T1-weighted fat-saturated image showing subtle enhancement in the thickened tibialis posterior tendon. (From Jakhere SG, Yadav D, Bharambay HV. Acute calcific tendinitis of tibialis posterior tendon (TPT): a rare site of involvement. *Eur J Radiol.* 2011;77(1):e17–e20 [Fig. 8]. ISSN 1571-4675, https://doi.org/10.1016/j.ejrex.2010.10.006, http://www.sciencedirect.com/science/article/pii/S1571467510 000799.)

The Science Behind the Diagnosis

ANATOMY OF THE POSTERIOR TIBIAL TENDON

The posterior tibialis muscle plantarflexes the foot at the ankle and inverts the foot at the subtalar and transverse tarsal joints. The muscle finds its origin from the posterior tibia and fibula. The tendon of the muscle passes behind the medial malleolus, running beneath the flexor retinaculum and into the sole of the foot, where it inserts on the navicular bone (Fig. 13.5). The posterior tibialis tendon is susceptible to the development of tendinitis where it curves around the medial malleolus.

CLINICAL SYNDROME

Posterior tibial tendinitis is being seen with increasing frequency in clinical practice as jogging and other aerobic exercises have increased in popularity. The posterior tibial tendon is susceptible to the development of tendinitis and is particularly subject to repetitive motion that may result in microtrauma,

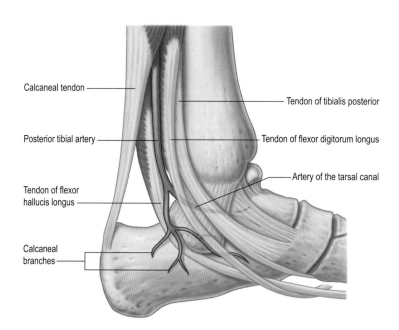

Fig. 13.5 Anatomy of the posterior tibial tendon. (From Standring S. *Gray's Anatomy: The Anatomic Basis of Clinical Practice*. ed. 42. Philadelphia: Elsevier; 2021 [Fig. 79-11].)

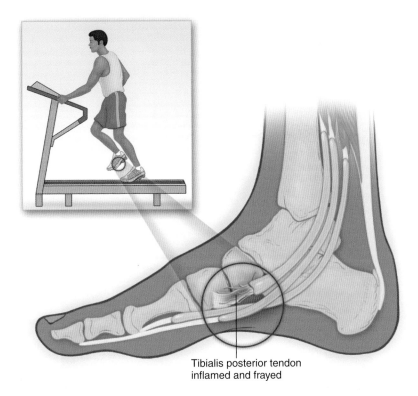

Tibialis posterior tendon
inflamed and frayed

Fig. 13.6 Running and high-impact aerobics routines are often implicated as inciting factors of acute posterior tibial tendinitis. (From Waldman S. *Atlas of Uncommon Pain Syndromes*. ed. 4. Philadelphia: Saunders; 2020 [Fig. 126-1].)

which heals poorly because of the tendon's avascularity. Running, Irish folk dancing, and high-impact aerobics routines are often implicated as inciting factors of acute posterior tibial tendinitis (Fig. 13.6). Tendinitis of the posterior tibial tendon frequently coexists with tendinitis of the Achilles tendon and bursitis of the associated bursa of the posterior ankle joint, creating additional pain and functional disability. Calcium deposition around the tendon may occur if the inflammation continues, making subsequent treatment more difficult (Fig. 13.7). Continued trauma to the inflamed tendon ultimately may result in tendon rupture (Fig. 13.8). In contrast to Achilles tendon rupture, which often occurs without warning after acute trauma, rupture of the posterior tibial tendon tends to be secondary to chronic tendinosis and degeneration of the tendon over time. Rupture of the posterior tibial tendon occurs three times more commonly in women, with peak incidence in the fifth and sixth decades. A left-sided predominance is seen, and rupture is unilateral more than 90% of the time.

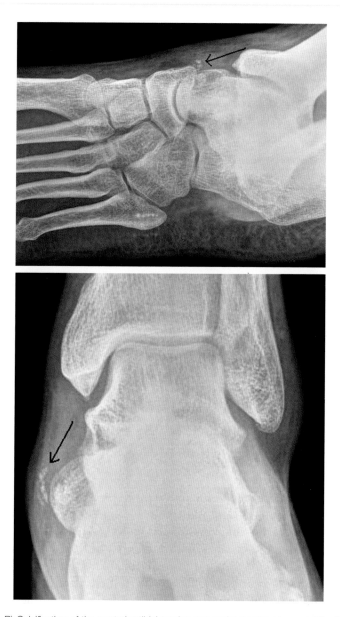

Fig. 13.7   (A, B) Calcification of the posterior tibial tendon can make treatment more difficult. Plain radiographs demonstrating calcification of the tendon in a patient suffering from posterior tibial tendinitis. (From Jakhere SG, Yadav D, Bharambay HV. Acute calcific tendinitis of tibialis posterior tendon (TPT): a rare site of involvement. *Eur J Radiol*. 2011;77(1):e17–e20 [Figs. 9 and 10]. ISSN 1571-4675, https://doi.org/10.1016/j.ejrex.2010.10.006, http://www.sciencedirect.com/science/article/pii/S1571467510000799.)

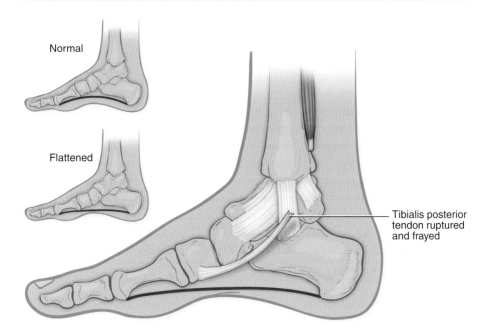

Fig. 13.8 Tendinitis of the posterior tibial tendon. Calcium deposition around the tendon may occur if the inflammation continues, making subsequent treatment more difficult. Continued trauma to the inflamed tendon ultimately may result in tendon rupture. (Modified from Waldman SD. *Atlas of Pain Management Injection Techniques*. ed. 3. Philadelphia: Saunders; 2013:353.)

SIGNS AND SYMPTOMS

The onset of posterior tibial tendinitis is usually gradual, occurring after overuse or misuse of the ankle joint. Inciting factors include activities such as running and sudden stopping and starting, as when playing tennis, or doing high-impact aerobics routines. Improper stretching of the gastrocnemius and tendons of the posterior ankle before exercise has been implicated in the development of posterior tibial tendinitis and acute tendon rupture. The pain of posterior tibial tendinitis is constant and severe and is localized over the medial longitudinal arch. Flattening of the medial longitudinal arch occurs, and over time a severe pes planus deformity results. Significant sleep disturbance is often reported. Weight bearing on the affected ankle and foot reveals these deformities and heel valgus, plantar flexion of the talus, and forefoot abduction. Patients with posterior tibial tendinitis or rupture, or both, exhibit weak inversion of the ankle and foot. A creaking or grating sensation may be palpated when passively plantar flexing and inverting the foot. Swelling and erythema over the inflamed tendon may be visible (see Fig. 13.1). As mentioned, the chronically inflamed posterior tibial tendon may rupture with stress or during vigorous injection procedures into the tendon itself.

TESTING

Plain radiographs, ultrasound imaging, and MRI are indicated for all patients with posterior ankle pain; weight-bearing radiographs often reveal the deformity associated with rupture of the posterior tibial tendon (Figs. 13.9, 13.10, 13.11, and 13.12; see Fig. 13.7). Based on the patient's clinical presentation, additional tests, including complete blood count, erythrocyte sedimentation rate, and antinuclear antibody testing, may be indicated. MRI of the ankle is indicated if joint instability is suspected. Radionuclide bone scanning identifies stress fractures of the tibia not seen on plain radiographs. Injection of the posterior tibial tendon with local anesthetic and steroid serves as a diagnostic and therapeutic maneuver (Fig. 13.13).

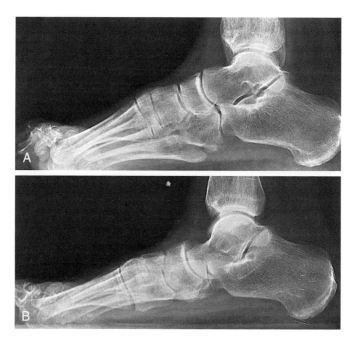

Fig. 13.9 Injuries of the tibialis posterior tendon: complete tears. Although a lateral radiograph obtained without weight bearing (A) appears normal, a lateral radiograph obtained with weight bearing (B) shows plantar flexion of the distal portion of the talus with malalignment at the talonavicular joint. (From Waldman SD. *Physical Diagnosis of Pain: An Atlas of Signs and Symptoms*. Philadelphia: Saunders; 2006:347.)

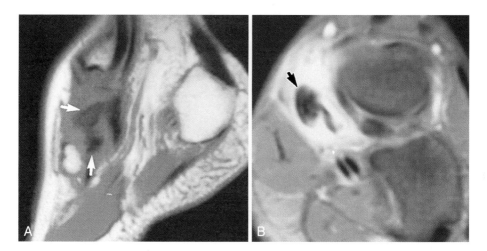

Fig. 13.10   Injuries of the tibialis posterior tendon: acute complete tear. (A) Sagittal T1-weighted (TR/TE, 800/12) spin echo magnetic resonance imaging (MRI) shows disorganization of the tibialis posterior tendon *(white arrows)* near its navicular site of insertion. Note a mass of intermediate signal intensity around the tendon. (B) Coronal T1-weighted (TR/TE, 650/20) spin echo MRI obtained with fat suppression after the intravenous administration of a gadolinium compound reveals the torn tibialis posterior tendon *(black arrow)*. Note the enhancement of signal intensity around the torn tendon. (From House CV, Connell DA, Saifuddin A. Posteromedial corner injuries of the knee. *Clin Radiol.* 2007;62:539–546.)

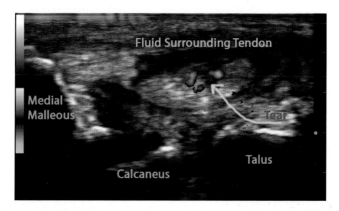

Fig. 13.11   Transverse color Doppler image demonstrating an acute tear of the tibialis posterior tendon. Note fluid surrounding the tendon.

DIFFERENTIAL DIAGNOSIS

Posterior tibial tendinitis generally is identified easily on clinical grounds. Because a bursa is located between the Achilles tendon and the base of the tibia

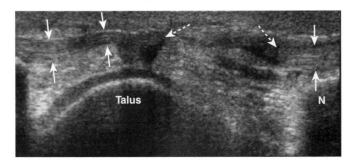

Fig. 13.12 Longitudinal ultrasound image of a complete rupture of the posterior tibial tendon. The proximal and distal tendon *(solid arrows)* is visualized inferior to the level of the medius malleolus, superficial to the talus, and inserting on the navicular *(N)*. The torn ends of the tendon *(broken arrows)* can be seen with some anechoic fluid within the tendon sheath. (From Waldman SD. Posterior tibial tendon rupture. In: Waldman SD, Campbell RSD, eds. *Imaging of Pain*. Philadelphia: Saunders; 2010:435−436.)

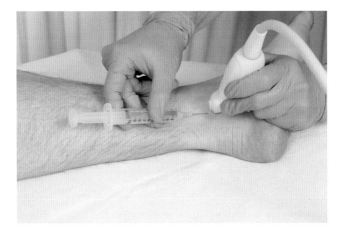

Fig. 13.13 Proper needle placement for an ultrasound-guided, in-plane injection for posterior tibialis tendinitis.

and the upper posterior calcaneus, coexistent bursitis may confuse the diagnosis. Stress fractures of the ankle and hindfoot may mimic posterior tibial tendinitis and may be identified on plain radiographs or radionuclide bone scanning.

TREATMENT

Initial treatment of the pain and functional disability associated with posterior tibial tendinitis should include a combination of nonsteroidal

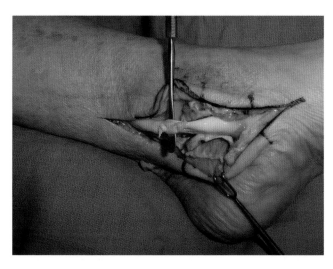

Fig. 13.14 Surgical exposure of the posterior tibial tendon. Note the significant tendinopathy. (From Pfeffer G, Easley M, Hintermann B, et al. *Operative Techniques: Foot and Ankle Surgery.* ed. 2. Philadelphia: Elsevier; 2018 [Fig. 30-3].)

antiinflammatory drugs or cyclooxygenase-2 inhibitors and physical therapy. Local application of heat and cold may be beneficial. The patient should be encouraged to avoid repetitive activities responsible for the evolution of the tendinitis, such as jogging. For patients with tendinitis of the posterior tibial tendon who do not respond to these treatment modalities, careful injection of the area underneath the deltoid ligament just below the medial malleolus with local anesthetic and steroid may be a reasonable next step (see Fig. 13.13). Surgery is required for patients who have sustained rupture of the posterior tibial tendon (Fig. 13.14).

HIGH-YIELD TAKEAWAYS

- The patient's symptomatology began after repeated jogging on a treadmill.
- The patient's pain is localized to the posterior tibial tendon.
- The patient is afebrile, making an acute infectious etiology unlikely.
- The lower extremity neurologic examination is within normal limits, making tarsal tunnel syndrome a likely diagnosis.
- X-ray of the posterior tibial tendon demonstrates characteristic findings, as does MRI and ultrasound imaging.

Suggested Readings

Bowring B, Chockalingam N. Conservative treatment of tibialis posterior tendon dysfunction—a review. *Foot*. 2010;20(1):18–26.

Noon M, Hoch AZ, McNamara L, et al. Injury patterns in female Irish dancers. *PM&R*. 2010;2(11):1030–1034.

Pedowitz D, Beck D. Presentation, diagnosis, and nonsurgical treatment options of the anterior tibial tendon, posterior tibial tendon, peroneals, and Achilles. *Foot Ankle Clin*. 2017;22(4):677–687.

Waldman SD. Posterior tibialis tendon injection. In: *Atlas of Pain Management Injection Techniques*. ed. 4. Philadelphia: Elsevier; 2017:658–660.

Waldman SD, Campbell RSD. Posterior tibial tendon rupture. In: *Imaging of Pain*. Philadelphia: Saunders; 2011:435–436.

Betty Bartholomew

A 32-Year-Old Pharmacist With Persistent Foot Pain

- Learn the common causes of foot pain.
- Develop an understanding of the unique vascular anatomy of the sesamoid.
- Develop an understanding of the causes of sesamoiditis.
- Learn the clinical presentation of sesamoiditis.
- Learn how to use physical examination to identify pathology of the sesamoid.
- Develop an understanding of the treatment options for sesamoiditis.
- Learn the appropriate testing options to help diagnose sesamoiditis.
- Learn to identify red flags in patients who present with foot pain.
- Develop an understanding of the role in interventional pain management in the treatment of sesamoiditis.

Betty Bartholomew

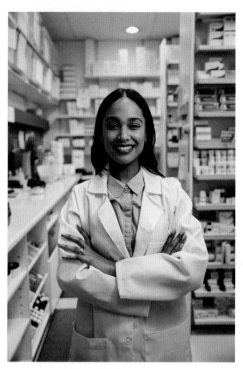

I entered the treatment room and sat down in front of my last patient and introduced myself. The young lady sitting in front of me looked familiar. As I was trying to remember where I had seen her, she must have noticed my perplexed look and stuck out her hand, saying, "My name is Betty Bartholomew. I work at the CVS Pharmacy on Main Street." I asked her, "So what brings you here today, Ms. Bartholomew?" She reported, "There is something seriously wrong with my right foot. I feel like I am standing on a stone. I looked it up on the Internet and it says I have a Morton neuroma, but I thought I better come in and get it checked out. My foot has been getting more painful in spite of everything I have tried: new shoes, a gelfoam mat to stand on, a Medrol Dosepak, Epsom salt soaks. Nothing seems to work. My friend, Kathy Brown, one of the other pharmacists, recommended you. She said you fixed her knee up after she feel on the ice getting out of the car last winter." I smiled and told her I was glad to hear that Kathy was doing well. Betty also noted that sometimes she used a heating pad, but she fell asleep with it on and accidently burned herself, so she was being really careful now to not use it as much.

I asked Betty if she had ever injured her foot before. She thought for a moment, then said, "No, I broke a finger when I slammed it in the car door about 10 years ago, but nothing with my feet. But, you know, foot pain is an occupational hazard for pharmacists. I stand all day long." Betty then volunteered that the only medication she is on is birth control pills.

I asked Betty to point with one finger to show me where it hurt the most. She pointed to the area at the head of the first metatarsal. "It feels like I'm stepping on a rock or something, and it really gets my attention whenever I stand for too long."

On physical examination, Betty was afebrile. Her respirations were 16. Her pulse was 68 and regular. Her blood pressure was normal at 112/76. Her head, eyes, ears, nose, throat (HEENT) exam was normal, as was her thyroid examination. Her cardiopulmonary examination was also normal, as was her abdominal examination, which revealed no abnormal mass or organomegaly. There was no

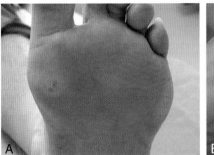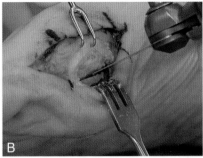

Fig. 14.1 (A) Clinical photograph of intractable plantar keratosis overlying an inflamed sesamoid bone. (B) Operative photograph demonstrating technique of sesamoid shaving. A saw is used to resect a portion of prominent sesamoid plantar surface. (From Cohen BE. Hallux sesamoid disorders. *Foot Ankle Clin.* 2009;14(1):91–104.)

costovertebral angle (CVA) tenderness. There was no peripheral edema. Her low back examination was unremarkable. Visual inspection of the radial aspect of the right foot revealed no cutaneous lesions or evidence of infection. There was no obvious bony deformity that would suggest a previous fracture. Nor were there any fibromas or plantar warts, but there was callus formation over the head of the first metatarsal (Fig. 14.1). The area overlying the head of the first metatarsal on the right was exquisitely tender to palpation. I had Betty flex and extend her big toe, and the tender area moved with the flexor tendon. Mulder sign was negative. The area was cool to touch. The left foot examination was normal, as was examination of her other major joints. A careful neurologic examination of the upper and lower extremities revealed no evidence of peripheral or entrapment neuropathy, and the deep tendon reflexes were normal.

Key Clinical Points—What's Important and What's Not

THE HISTORY

- History of increasing right foot pain with the sensation of standing on a stone
- An increase in pain with weight bearing
- An increase in pain with prolonged standing
- No history of previous trauma to the right foot
- No fever or chills

THE PHYSICAL EXAMINATION

- Patient is afebrile
- Callus formation over the head of the first metatarsal on the right

- Palpation of area overlying the head of the first metatarsal on the right elicits sharp pain
- The painful area moves with the flexor tendon, which is highly suggestive of sesamoiditis
- Mulder sign is negative

OTHER FINDINGS OF NOTE

- Normal blood pressure
- Normal HEENT examination
- Normal cardiovascular examination
- Normal pulmonary examination
- Normal abdominal examination
- No peripheral edema
- No CVA tenderness
- Normal upper extremity neurologic examination, motor and sensory examination

 ## What Tests Would You Like to Order?

The following tests were ordered:
- Plain radiograph of the right foot with special attention to the metatarsal heads
- Computed tomography (CT) scan of the right foot with special attention to the sesamoid bones

TEST RESULTS

The plain radiographs of the right foot revealed an apparent stress fracture of the tibial sesamoid with diastasis (Fig. 14.2).

CT of the right foot revealed fragmentation and sclerosis of the tibial sesamoid (Fig. 14.3).

 ## Clinical Correlation—Putting it all Together

What is the diagnosis?
- Sesamoiditis with stress fracture of the tibial sesamoid bone

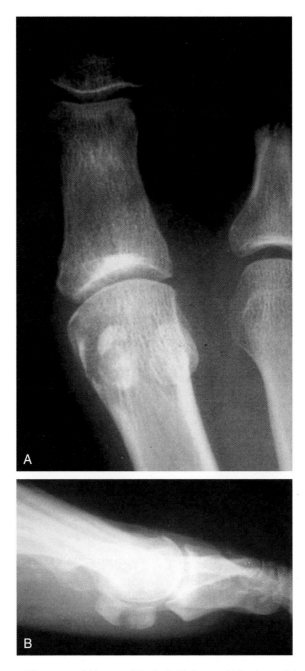

Fig. 14.2 Fractures of the sesamoid bones of the foot. (A) Sesamoid fractures. Anteroposterior radiograph of stress fracture of tibial sesamoid with diastasis. (B) Lateral radiograph of stress fracture of tibial sesamoid with diastasis. (From Cohen BE. Hallux sesamoid disorders. *Foot Ankle Clin.* 2009;14 (1):91–104.)

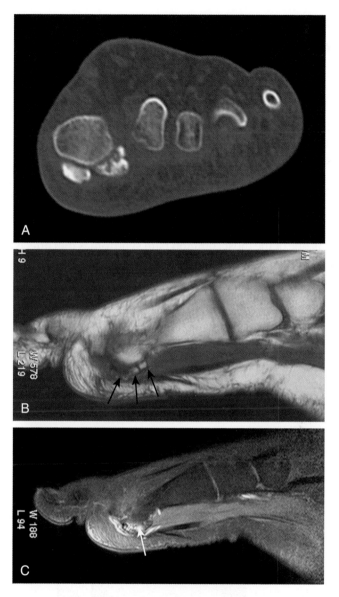

Fig. 14.3 (A) Coronal computerized tomography scan of a patient with sesamoiditis, demonstrating fragmentation and sclerosis of the lateral sesamoid. (B) The sagittal T1-weighted (T1W) magnetic resonance imaging (MRI) also demonstrates the bony fragmentation *(black arrows)*. (C) High-signal intensity reactive edema is present on the corresponding fat-suppressed T2W MRI *(white arrow)*. (From Waldman SD, Campbell RSD. *Imaging of Pain*. Philadelphia, Elsevier; 2011.)

The Science Behind the Diagnosis

ANATOMY

The sesamoid bones are small, rounded structures that are embedded in the flexor tendons of the foot and usually are in close proximity to the joints. Sesamoid bones of the first metatarsal occur in almost all patients, with sesamoid bones being present in the flexor tendons of the second and fifth metatarsals in a significant number of patients (Fig. 14.4). These sesamoid bones serve to decrease friction and pressure of the flexor tendon as it passes in proximity to a joint.

CLINICAL PRESENTATION

Sesamoiditis is one of the most common pain syndromes that affects the forefoot. It is characterized by tenderness and pain over the metatarsal heads. Although the first sesamoid bone of the first metatarsal head is affected most commonly, the sesamoid bones of the second and fifth metatarsal heads also are subject to the development of sesamoiditis. Patients often report it feels like they are walking with a stone in their shoe (Fig. 14.5). The pain of sesamoiditis worsens with prolonged standing or walking for long distances and is exacerbated by improperly fitting or padded shoes. Sesamoiditis is most often associated with pushing-off injuries during football or repetitive microtrauma from running or dancing. These sesamoid bones decrease friction and pressure of the flexor tendon as it passes in proximity to a joint.

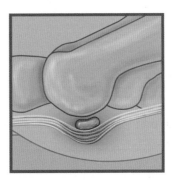

Fig. 14.4 The sesamoid bones are small, rounded structures that are embedded in the flexor tendons of the foot and usually are in close proximity to the joints. Sesamoid bones of the first metatarsal occur in almost all patients, with sesamoid bones being present in the flexor tendons of the second and fifth metatarsals in a significant number of patients. (From Waldman S. *Atlas of Pain Management Injection Techniques*. ed. 4. St. Louis: Elsevier; 2017 [Fig. 181-1].)

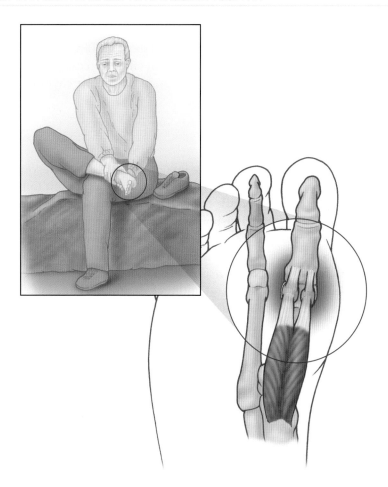

Fig. 14.5 Patients with sesamoiditis often feel like they are walking with a stone in their shoe. (From Waldman S. *Atlas of Common Pain Syndromes*. ed. 4. Philadelphia: Elsevier; 2019 [Fig. 134-1].)

SIGNS AND SYMPTOMS

The patient suffering from sesamoiditis will experience pain with any weight bearing that worsens with prolonged standing and walking. Stair climbing may become increasingly difficult as the inflammation increases. Wearing high heels, poorly fitting, and/or inadequately padded shoes will exacerbate the patient's functional disability and pain. Often, the patient with sesamoiditis will experience the sensation of walking on a stone in the shoe.

On physical examination, pain can be reproduced by pressure on the sesamoid bone. In contradistinction to metatarsalgia, in which the tender area remains over the metatarsal heads, with sesamoiditis, the tender area moves with the flexor tendon when the patient actively flexes the toe. A callus overlying the affected sesamoid bone may be present (see Fig. 14.1). The patient with sesamoiditis often exhibits an antalgic gait in an effort to reduce weight bearing during walking. With acute trauma to the sesamoid bone, ecchymosis over the plantar surface of the foot may be present.

TESTING

Plain radiographs, magnetic resonance imaging (MRI), and ultrasound imaging are indicated in all patients who present with pain thought to be caused by sesamoiditis to rule out occult bony disorders and tumor (Fig. 14.6; see Figs. 14.2 and 14.3). Radionuclide bone scanning may rule out stress fractures not visible on plain radiographs (Fig. 14.7). Based on the patient's clinical presentation, additional testing may be warranted, including a complete blood count, comprehensive metabolic profile, prostate-specific antigen level, erythrocyte sedimentation rate, and antinuclear antibody testing. The injection technique described later serves as both a diagnostic and a therapeutic maneuver.

DIFFERENTIAL DIAGNOSIS

Morton neuroma and intermetatarsal bursitis are often confused with the inflammation and fractures of the sesamoid bones of the foot (Fig. 14.8), although the pain of sesamoid fracture is localized to the plantar surface of the foot and is less neuritic than that of Morton neuroma. Tendinitis and metatarsal stress fractures of the foot can also mimic the pain of Morton neuroma.

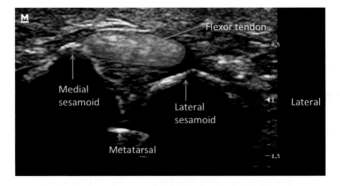

Fig. 14.6 Ultrasound image demonstrating the lateral and medial sesamoids overlying the metatarsals. (From Waldman S. *Atlas of Common Pain Syndromes*. ed. 4. Philadelphia: Elsevier; 2019 [Fig. 134-5].)

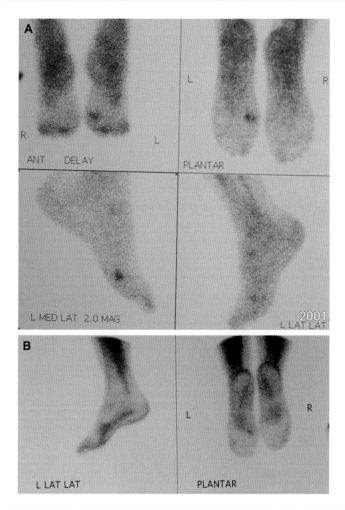

Fig. 14.7 (A, B) Sesamoiditis. Technetium-99 bone scan with localized views of the forefoot demonstrating sesamoiditis. (From Waldman S. *Atlas of Common Pain Syndromes*. ed. 4. Philadelphia: Elsevier; 2019 [Fig. 134-6].)

TREATMENT

Initial treatment of the pain and functional disability associated with sesamoiditis includes a combination of nonsteroidal antiinflammatory drugs (NSAIDs) or cyclooxygenase-2 inhibitors and physical therapy. The local application of heat and cold may also be beneficial. Avoidance of repetitive activities that aggravate the patient's symptoms, avoidance of walking barefoot or with shoes that do not provide good support, and short-term immobilization of the affected foot may provide relief. For patients who do not respond to these treatment modalities, injection with local anesthetic and steroid is a reasonable next step (Fig. 14.9).

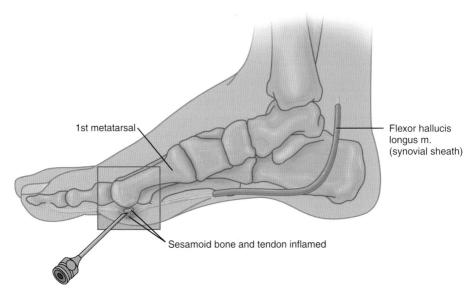

Fig. 14.8 Proper needle position for sesamoid bone injection of the foot. (From Waldman SD. *Atlas of Pain Management Injection Techniques*. ed. 5. Philadelphia, Elsevier; 2017:680.)

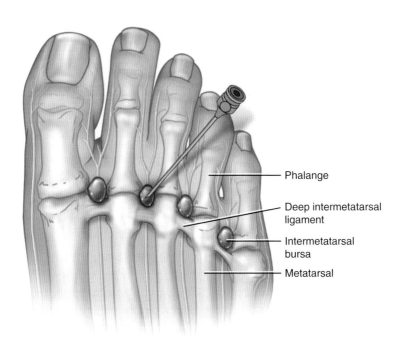

Fig. 14.9 Intermetatarsal bursitis can mimic the pain of sesamoiditis. (From Waldman S. *Atlas of Pain Management Injection Techniques*. ed. 4. St. Louis: Elsevier; 2017 [Fig. 180-5].)

Physical modalities, including local heat and gentle stretching exercises, should be introduced several days after the patient undergoes injection. Vigorous exercises should be avoided because they will exacerbate the patient's symptoms. Metatarsal pads or molded orthotic devices may also be of value. Simple analgesics, NSAIDs, and antimyotonic agents, such as tizanidine, can be used concurrently with this injection technique.

HIGH-YIELD TAKEAWAYS

- The patient is afebrile, making an acute infectious etiology (e.g., septic arthritis) unlikely.
- The history of the sensation of feeling like one is standing on a stone is suggestive of the diagnosis of Morton neuroma or sesamoiditis.
- The patient's pain is highly localized and moves with the flexor tendon, which is highly suggestive of sesamoiditis.
- The patient's symptoms are unilateral and involve only one joint, which is more suggestive of a local process than a systemic polyarthropathy.
- Plain radiographs and CT will provide high-yield information regarding the bony contents of the joint, but ultrasound imaging and MRI will be more useful in identifying soft tissue pathology.
- Bone scan may be useful in identifying fracture or sesamoiditis not seen on x-ray.

Suggested Readings

Cohen BE. Hallux sesamoid disorders. *Foot Ankle Clin*. 2009;14(1):91–104.

Kulemann V, Mayerhoefer M, Trnka HJ, et al. Abnormal findings in hallucal sesamoids on MR imaging—associated with different pathologies of the forefoot? An observational study. *Eur J Radiol*. 2010;74(1):226–230.

Schein AJ, Skalski MR, Patel DB, et al. Turf toe and sesamoiditis: what the radiologist needs to know. *Clin Imaging*. 2015;39(3):380–389.

Waldman SD. Injection technique for sesamoiditis pain. In: *Atlas of Pain Management Injection Techniques*. ed. 4. Philadelphia: Elsevier; 2017:678–681.

Waldman SD. Sesamoiditis. In: *Waldman's Comprehensive Atlas of Diagnostic Ultrasound of Painful Conditions*. Philadelphia: Wolters Kluwer; 2016:1179–1186.

Waldman SD, Campbell RSD. Sesamoiditis. In: *Imaging of Pain*. Philadelphia: Saunders; 2011:455–456.

Chuck North

A 32-Year-Old Veteran With Pain in the Ball of His Foot

- Learn the common causes of foot pain.
- Develop an understanding of the anatomy of the metatarsals.
- Develop an understanding of the causes of metatarsalgia.
- Develop an understanding of the differential diagnosis of foot pain.
- Learn the clinical presentation of metatarsalgia.
- Learn how to use physical examination to identify metatarsalgia.
- Develop an understanding of the treatment options for metatarsalgia.

Chuck North

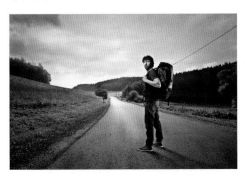

Chuck North is a 32-year-old veteran with the chief complaint of, "The bottom of my foot hurts." Chuck stated that over the last couple of months, he has been experiencing increasing pain on the ball of his right foot. He went on to say that it came on gradually since he began his cross-country trek that he started on Veterans Day last year. "Doc, I know I look like 10 miles of bad road, but the Army taught me how to take care of my feet, and I have been very careful about that. But I am barely making it 20 miles a day with this foot pain. A veterans group in Kansas City gave me some new shoes, and I thought that would help, but it really didn't."

Chuck noted that the pain got a little better when he got off his feet, but walking was making the pain much worse. He figured that if he took it a little easier that he would get better over time, but it just didn't happen. Walking became a real problem, as did any weight bearing. He tried to elevate his feet at night, which provided only minimal relief. He used Extra-Strength Tylenol when he could get it, which he felt took the edge off. "Doctor, please help me. I need to complete this walk to honor my buddies who didn't make it back."

I asked Chuck if he had experienced any foot pain in the past, and he replied, "Never. Doc, like I said, even if I am between places to stay, I take good care of my feet. You know it's not true that an army moves on its stomach. An army moves on its feet. You can do okay if you miss a few meals, but let me tell you, you are in trouble if your feet hurt! Ask any GI and they will tell you the same thing: Take care of your feet."

I asked Chuck how he was sleeping, and he said, "Not worth a crap, Doc. I haven't slept that well since I rotated out, but this foot hurts 24/7. Every time I roll over, the pain wakes me up. The biggest problem is that I can't walk for more than a few minutes without the pain playing up. It really slows me down. Walking has become a real problem. I try to hitchhike, but that kind of defeats the purpose."

I asked Chuck to show me where the pain was, and he pointed to the area over his right metatarsal heads. "Doc, this is right where the pain is. Most of the time I feel like I have something in my shoe, like a rock or something. I bet I empty my shoes 100 times a day. There is rarely anything to dump out." I asked, "Does the pain radiate anywhere?" Chuck shook his head and said, "It's just the ball of my right foot. It is sore all of the time. I must have broken it or something. In the Army, there was a thing called a march fracture, although it's been a while since I marched. Does walking across country count?" I asked Chuck about any fever, chills, or other constitutional symptoms such as weight loss or night sweats, and he shook his head no. He denied any musculoskeletal, systemic symptoms, or bowel or bladder symptoms.

On physical examination, Chuck was afebrile. His respirations were 18, his pulse was 72 and regular, and his blood pressure was 124/76. Chuck's head, eyes, ears, nose, throat (HEENT) exam was normal, as was his thyroid exam. Auscultation of his carotids revealed no bruits, and the pulses in all four extremities were normal. He had a regular rhythm without ectopy. His cardiac exam was otherwise unremarkable. His abdominal examination revealed no abnormal mass or organomegaly. There was no peripheral edema. His low back examination was unremarkable. There was no costovertebral angle (CVA) tenderness. Visual inspection of his right foot revealed a callus over the metatarsal heads (Fig. 15.1). Otherwise, the skin over his metatarsal heads was unremarkable. Specifically, there was no rubor or calor, and there was no evidence of ecchymosis or anything suggestive of plantar warts. Palpation of the metatarsal heads caused Chuck to cry out in pain. "Doc, you're right on it! Please don't push that hard! I have had about all the fun I want to with that, enough already!" A careful

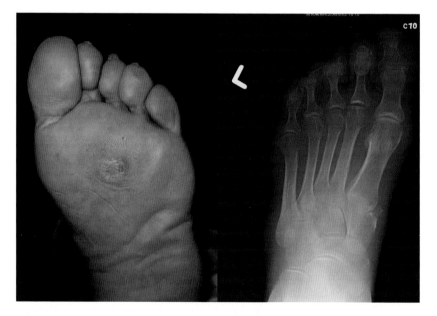

Fig. 15.1 A case of metatarsalgia with callosity underneath the third metatarsal head *(left)*. X-rays showed no discrepancy in the metatarsal length *(right)*. (From Lui TH. Percutaneous dorsal closing wedge osteotomy of the metatarsal neck in management of metatarsalgia. *Foot*. 2014;24(4):180–185 [Fig. 1]. ISSN 0958-2592, https://doi.org/10.1016/j.foot.2014.08.008, http://www.sciencedirect.com/science/article/pii/S0958259214000790.)

neurologic examination of both lower extremities was within normal limits, specifically there was no evidence of tarsal tunnel syndrome. I had Chuck wiggle his big toe on the right and the pain stayed localized, making the diagnosis of sesamoiditis less likely. Mulder sign was negative. Deep tendon reflexes were physiologic throughout.

Key Clinical Points—What's Important and What's Not

THE HISTORY

- History of onset of severe pain in the ball of the foot after prolonged walking
- Pain is localized to the metatarsal heads
- Any activities that cause pressure of the metatarsal heads cause pain
- Significant sleep disturbance
- No fever or chills

THE PHYSICAL EXAMINATION

- Patient is afebrile
- Marked tenderness to palpation of the metatarsal heads
- Callus formation over the metatarsal heads on the right (see Fig. 15.1)
- Pain remains localized over the metatarsal heads when the patient flexes and extends toes
- Palpation of the metatarsal heads did not reveal any obvious bony deformity or abnormal mass
- No evidence of plantar warts (Fig. 15.2)
- Normal neurologic examination

OTHER FINDINGS OF NOTE

- Normal HEENT examination
- Normal cardiovascular examination
- Normal pulmonary examination
- Normal abdominal examination
- No peripheral edema

What Tests Would You Like to Order?

The following tests were ordered:
- X-ray of the foot

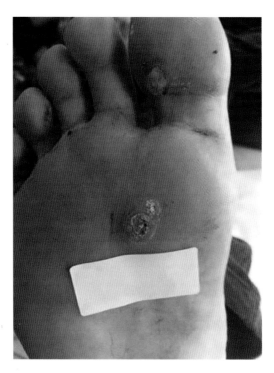

Fig. 15.2 Myrmecia (plantar) warts appear as rough, horny elevations on the plantar surface. They are caused by human papillomavirus type I.

TEST RESULTS

X-ray of the foot revealed a pes cavus deformity with a high calcaneal pitch. No fracture is noted (Fig. 15.3).

Clinical Correlation—Putting it all Together

What is the diagnosis?
- Metatarsalgia

The Science Behind the Diagnosis

ANATOMY

The strength of the foot is based on the arch-type configuration of the bones and ligaments (Fig. 15.4). This configuration gives the foot an amazing amount of strength and resiliency during the stresses of weight bearing and walking.

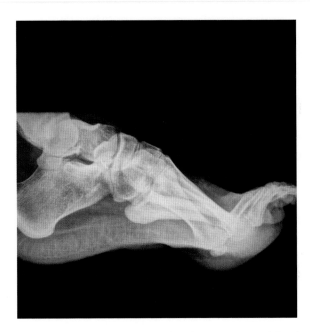

Fig. 15.3 X-ray of a patient with metatarsalgia demonstrating a pes cavus deformity displaying a high calcaneal pitch leading to a rigid foot type often predisposed to a tight Achilles tendon and metatarsalgia.

Anything that alters the structural integrity of the arches or changes the way that stresses are applied to these arches usually results in pain and disability and may cause callus formation (Fig. 15.5). The first metatarsal bone is similar to the first metacarpal in that it is not connected to the second metatarsal by any ligaments. The bases of the other four metatarsal bones are attached to one another by the dorsal, plantar, and interosseous ligaments. The heads of the metatarsal bones are connected via the transverse metatarsal ligaments. The transverse metatarsal ligament is subject to strain, especially in long-distance runners, that may coexist with metatarsalgia. Sesamoid bones beneath the heads of the metatarsal bones are present in some individuals and are subject to the development of inflammation. The muscles of the metatarsal joints and their attaching tendons are susceptible to trauma and to wear and tear from overuse and misuse.

CLINICAL SYNDROME

Along with sesamoiditis, metatarsalgia is another painful condition of the forefoot being seen with increasing frequency in clinical practice because of the increased interest in jogging and long-distance running. Metatarsalgia is characterized by tenderness and pain over the metatarsal heads. Patients often feel they

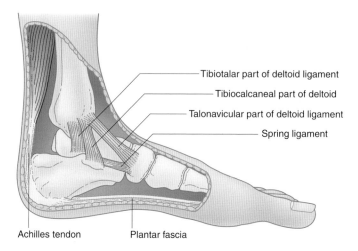

Fig. 15.4 The arch of the foot. (From Waldman S. *Pain Review*. ed. 2. Philadelphia: Elsevier; 2017 [Fig. 91-1].)

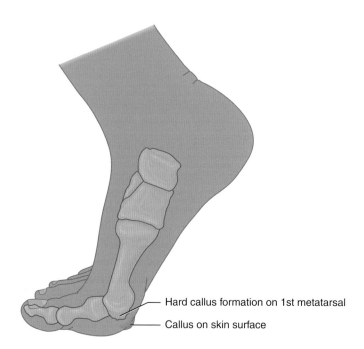

Fig. 15.5 Plantar keratosis (callus) over the metatarsal heads is the result of the patient attempting to shift pressure off the painful head of the first metatarsal to the heads of the second and third metatarsals. (From Waldman S. *Atlas of Pain Management Injection Techniques*. ed. 4. St. Louis: Elsevier; 2017 [Fig. 182-1].)

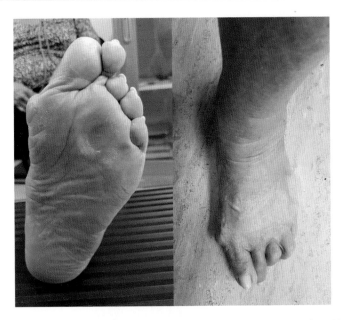

Fig. 15.6 Plantar keratosis over the metatarsal heads in a patient with metatarsalgia, Note the hallux valgus and hammertoe deformities. (From Negrín FV. Metatarsalgia. *FMC*. 2020;27(3):139—144 [Fig. 1]. ISSN 1134-2072, https://doi.org/10.1016/j.fmc.2019.10.008, http://www.sciencedirect.com/science/article/pii/S1134207219302397.)

are walking with a stone in their shoe. The pain of metatarsalgia worsens with prolonged standing or walking for long distances and is exacerbated by improperly fitting or padded shoes. Often, a patient with metatarsalgia develops a hard callus over the heads of the second and third metatarsals from trying to shift the weight off the head of the first metatarsal to relieve the pain (Fig. 15.6). This callus increases the pressure on the metatarsal heads and exacerbates the patient's pain and disability.

SIGNS AND SYMPTOMS

On physical examination, pain can be reproduced by pressure on the metatarsal heads (Fig. 15.7). Callus often is present over the heads of the second and third metatarsal heads and can be distinguished from plantar warts by the lack of thrombosed blood vessels that appear as small dark spots through the substance of the wart when the surface is trimmed (see Fig. 15.2). A patient with metatarsalgia often exhibits an antalgic gait in an effort to reduce weight bearing during the static stance phase of walking. Ligamentous laxity and flattening of the transverse arch also may be present, giving the foot a splayed-out appearance.

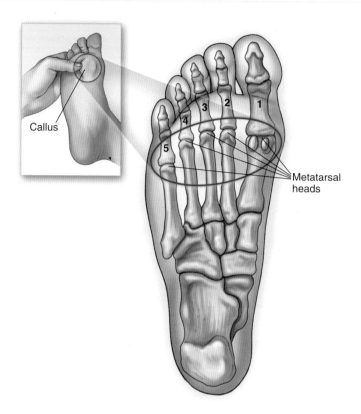

Fig. 15.7 On physical examination, pain can be reproduced by pressure on the metatarsal heads. (From Waldman S. *Atlas of Uncommon Pain Syndromes*. ed. 4. Philadelphia: Saunders; 2020 [Fig. 134-1].)

TESTING

Plain radiographs are indicated in all patients with metatarsalgia to rule out fractures and to identify sesamoid bones that may have become inflamed (Figs. 15.8, 15.9, and 15.10). Based on the patient's clinical presentation, additional tests, including complete blood cell count, erythrocyte sedimentation rate, and antinuclear antibody testing, may be indicated. Magnetic resonance imaging (MRI), computer tomography scanning, and ultrasound imaging of the metatarsal bones is indicated if joint instability, occult mass, or tumor is suspected (Figs. 15.11 and 15.12). Radionucleotide bone scanning may be useful in identifying stress fractures that may be missed on plain radiographs of the foot.

DIFFERENTIAL DIAGNOSIS

Primary pathology of the foot, including gout and occult fractures, may mimic the pain and disability associated with metatarsalgia. Entrapment neuropathies

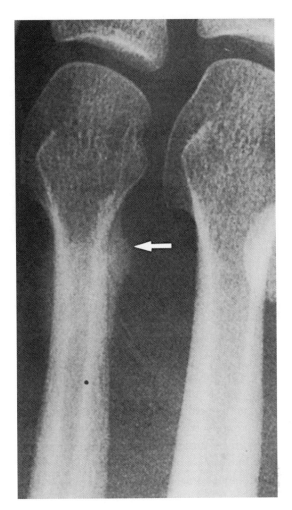

Fig. 15.8 Stress fracture of the metatarsal ("march fracture"). Anteroposterior radiograph shows fluffy periosteal new bone along the distal shaft of the third metatarsal *(arrow);* the patient had foot pain for 16 days. (From Grainger RG, Allison D. *Grainger and Allison's Diagnostic Radiology: A Textbook of Medical Imaging.* ed. 3. New York: Churchill Livingstone; 1997:1610.)

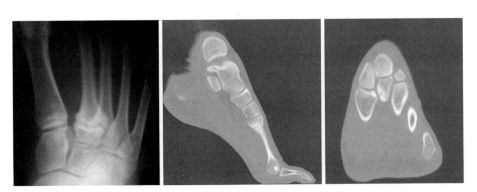

Fig. 15.9 Stress fracture of the base of the second metatarsal in dancers. Radiographic anterior (left image)-posterior (center image) view and computed tomography scan (right image), sagittal and transverse plane views, demonstrating the transverse fracture line. (From Porter D, Schon L. *Baxter's the Foot and Ankle in Sport.* ed. 3. Elsevier; 2020:255-274 [Fig. 24-11].)

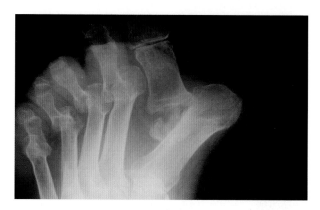

Fig. 15.10   A rheumatoid foot with associated severe deformities, including dislocation of metatarso-phalangeal joints leading to metatarsalgia due to increased pressures. (From Chahal GS, Davies MB, Blundell CM. Treating metatarsalgia: current concepts. *Orthop Trauma*. 2020;34(1):30−36 [Fig. 4]. ISSN 1877-1327, https://doi.org/10.1016/j.mporth.2019.11.005, http://www.sciencedirect.com/science/article/pii/S1877132719301265.)

such as tarsal tunnel syndrome, bursitis, and plantar fasciitis of the foot also may confuse the diagnosis; bursitis and plantar fasciitis may coexist with sesamoiditis. Sesamoid bones beneath the heads of the metatarsal bones are present in some individuals and are subject to the development of inflammation termed sesamoiditis. Sesamoiditis is another common cause of forefoot pain and may be distinguished from metatarsalgia by the fact that the pain of metatarsalgia is centered over the patient's metatarsal heads and does not move when the patient actively flexes the toes, as is the case with sesamoiditis. The muscles of the metatarsal joints and their attaching tendons are susceptible to trauma and wear and tear from overuse and misuse and may contribute to forefoot pain. Primary and metastatic tumors of the foot also may manifest in a manner analogous to that of arthritis of the midtarsal joints.

TREATMENT

Initial treatment of the pain and functional disability associated with metatarsalgia should include a combination of nonsteroidal antiinflammatory drugs or cyclooxygenase-2 inhibitors and physical therapy. Local application of heat and cold may be beneficial. Avoidance of repetitive activities that aggravate the patient's symptoms and short-term immobilization of the midtarsal joint also may provide relief. For patients who do not respond to these treatment modalities, injection of the affected metatarsal heads with a local anesthetic and steroid may be a reasonable next step (Fig. 15.13). Rocker-bottom shoes may also provide relief (Fig. 15.14).

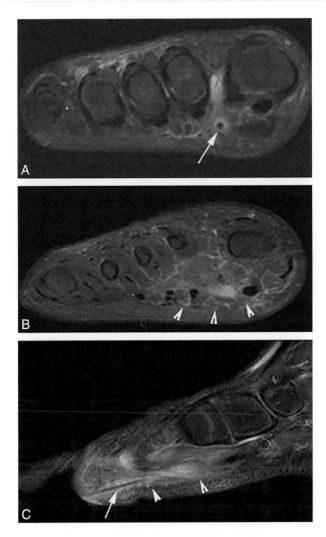

Fig. 15.11 Forefoot foreign-body granuloma. A 35-year-old agricultural worker presented with 1-month history of metatarsalgia with unclear traumatic history. Proton density fat-saturated short-axis images (A, B) and sagittal image (C) showed a thin signal-void structure that is linear on sagittal image and rounded on short-axis images. It is surrounded by hyperintense halo and hyperintense signal of the surrounding soft tissues of the plantar aspect of first intermetatarsal space. A palm thorn was retrieved on surgical exploration. (From Nouh MR, El-Gawad EAA, Abdulsalam SM. MRI utility in patients with non-traumatic metatarsalgia: a tertiary musculoskeletal center observational study. *Egypt J Radiol Nuclear Med*. 2015;46(4):1057–1064 [Fig. 5].)

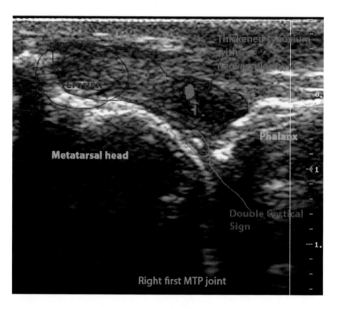

Fig. 15.12 Ultrasound image demonstrating gout involving the metatarsophalangeal joint. Note the double cortical sign.

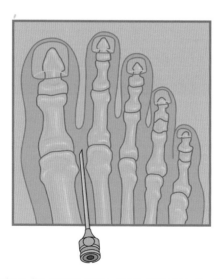

Fig. 15.13 Injection technique for metatarsalgia. (From Waldman S. *Atlas of Pain Management Injection Techniques*. ed. 4. St. Louis: Elsevier; 2017 [Fig. 182-3].)

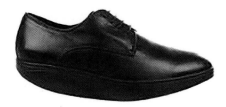

Fig. 15.14   Rocker-bottom shoes may help take the pressure off the metatarsal heads.

HIGH-YIELD TAKEAWAYS

- The patient is afebrile, making an acute infectious etiology unlikely.
- The patient's symptomatology is most likely due to microtrauma to the metatarsal heads from long-distance walking.
- Physical examination and testing should focus on identification of other pathologic processes that may mimic the clinical diagnosis of metatarsalgia.
- The patient exhibits physical examination findings that are highly suggestive of metatarsalgia.
- The patient's symptoms are localized.
- Plain radiographs of the metatarsal heads will help identify bony abnormalities of the metatarsal heads, including fractures, dislocations, and osseous tumors.
- Ultrasound imaging, computed tomography scanning, and MRI of the metatarsal heads may help identify less common causes of foot pain.

Suggested Readings

Chahal GS, Davies MB, Blundell CM. Treating metatarsalgia: current concepts. *Orthop Trauma*. 2020;34(1):30–36.

Gregg JM, Schneider T, Marks P. MR imaging and ultrasound of metatarsalgia—the lesser metatarsals. *Radiol Clin N Am*. 2008;46(6):1061–1078.

Hodes A, Umans H. Metatarsalgia. *Radiol Clin N Am*. 2018;56(6):877–892.

Klammer G, Espinosa N. Scientific evidence in the treatment of metatarsalgia. *Foot Ankle Clin*. 2019;24(4):585–598.

Waldman SD. Metatarsalgia. In: *Atlas of Uncommon Pain Syndromes*. ed. 4. Philadelphia: Elsevier; 2021:452–453.

Note: Page numbers followed by 'f' indicate figures; those followed by 't' indicate tables and 'b' indicate boxes

L

Lumbar radiculopathy, 10–11,
61–62
Lyme disease, 7, 11*f*

M

Matles test, for Achilles tendon
rupture, 100*f*
Medial ankle
instability, rotatory drawer
testing, 35–36, 37*f*
ligaments of, 40*f*
pain. *See* Ankle pain, medial
Medial plantar proper digital
nerve (MPPDN), 138*f*
Metatarsal bone, 218–219
Metatarsalgia, 209–210, 216*f*,
219–221
Metatarsal stress fractures,
210
Metatarsophalangeal joint
osteoarthritis of, 132*f*
of toes, anatomy, 132–133,
133*f*, 146, 147*f*
ultrasound-guided out-of-
plane injection of, 139*f*
Midtarsal joints
arthritis of, 26, 29–31
Charcot, 26
Charcot neuroarthropathy of,
26, 26*f*
Morton neuroma, 158–160,
161*f*, 210
digital nerve stretch test for,
156*f*
Mulder sign for, 156*f*

Morton neuroma (*Continued*)
needle placement for
injection of, 165*f*
surgical extirpation of, 166*f*
MPPDN. *See* Medial plantar
proper digital nerve
(MPPDN)
Myrmecia (plantar) warts,
218*f*

N

Neuroma, Joplin, 136–137,
138*f*
Neuroma, Morton, 158–160,
161*f*, 210
digital nerve stretch test for,
156*f*
Mulder sign for, 156*f*
needle placement for
injection of, 165*f*
surgical extirpation of, 166*f*
Neuropathies, entrapment,
10–11, 222–224
Nonsteroidal antiinflammatory
drugs (NSAIDs),
45–49, 93–94

O

Obesity, 174, 177*f*
Osteoarthritis, 7, 13*f*, 23, 26,
116–117, 117*f*
of ankle and subtalar joint,
55*f*
of metatarsophalangeal joint,
132*f*